IO TEARS LEFT

DOM COLBERT

ABOUT THE AUTHOR

Dr Dom Colbert has worked as a volunteer in developing countries since 1960. He worked in many disaster areas, including Biafra, Ethiopia and Bosnia to mention but a few. He is currently an honorary Senior Clinical Lecturer in the Department of International Health and Tropical Medicine in the Royal College of Surgeons, Dublin, and an Invited Lecturer in Tropical Medicine in National University of Ireland Galway (NUIG), where he taught Applied Physiology for many years.

He has lectured widely in Europe and the United States and has written extensively on medical topics. He was part of the Executive Committee of Medicus Mundi International in 1991 that was honoured with the Prince of Asturias Award for the development of healthcare in deprived countries and in 2013 he was made a Fellow of the College of Surgeons of East, Central and Southern Africa for 'outstanding service to surgery in Africa'. He lives in Galway, Ireland.

NO TEARS LEFT

BIAFRA TO BOSNIA

Further Memories of an Irish Doctor Abroad

DOM COLBERT

ORPEN PRESS

Published by
Orpen Press
Upper Floor, Unit K9
Greenogue Business Park
Rathcoole
Co. Dublin
Ireland
email: info@orpenpress.com
www.orpenpress.com

ISBN 978-1-78605-056-4

Printed in Dublin by SPRINTprint Ltd

To all those, known and unknown, who have given their time and sometimes their lives in the service of the less fortunate at home or overseas, and to those who have supported them down the years.

ACKNOWLEDGEMENTS

I could never have written this account of my 'hidden life' without the encouragement and patience of my late wife, Doreen, and of our five children, Mary, Sallyann, Sibylline, Danielle and Serryth. Much of their young lives was spent in wondering where I was and when – and if – I would return. Many friends, colleagues and past students have encouraged me to put this account on paper, none more so than Professor Ger O'Flaherty of Galway, who may someday write his own account of working in foreign lands. I also thank Fr Tom Jordan OP for allowing me to use the incident of the Prophet David which appeared in *Spirituality* a few years ago. A special word of thanks goes to the Royal College of Surgeons in Dublin and in particular to Professor Sam McConkey and to the Dean of Medicine in Galway, Prof Tim O'Brien for immediate and unquestioned support. Finally, I want to thank the Medical Missionary of Mary Sisters Isabelle Smyth, Deirdre Twomey and Carla Simmons for correcting my memory on so many occasions, Conail O'Cuinn for his comments on my work and everyone in Orpen Press, especially the commissioning editor Ailbhe O'Reilley who believed in my work from the start, as well as the senior editor Eileen Obrien and Gerry Kelly for their support and forbearance at all times.

CONTENTS

PREFACE

I wrote most of this book as I sat beside my wife Doreen when she was receiving chemotherapy. She had always wanted to know about the 'other half' of my life, that half when I had left her and the children at home in Ireland to work as a doctor in some of the wars and famines that have plagued our times.

I promised to let her read it as soon as it was finished. Sadly, that day never came. But I still feel that I should share it with others, for it is an account of a life riddled with small successes and failures, in which any of us could have been the principal actor.

Everything I have written is true *as far as my memory permits*. If I have hurt anybody, I sincerely apologise, for no hurt was intended. If I have failed to acknowledge anyone who has helped me during my life, I apologise too, for such omissions are also unintentional.

In some places, I have changed names and slightly altered the chronology so that the narrative can run more smoothly. However, I have not purposefully altered the facts.

Finally, I warn you not to look for anything more than what I tell, or you may be disappointed, for it is a simple story that carries no great philosophical message. I merely invite the reader to share my experience of life and make her or his own judgment.

Dom Colbert
Galway, Ireland, 2018

CHAPTER 1

TIME TO GO

The Call of the Coast

In July 1967, military hostilities began between the small breakaway state of Biafra and the rest of Nigeria. Technically, this was a civil war, but some saw it as a battle for the survival of the Igbos. It was a David versus Goliath contest, but this time there would be no fairy-tale ending.

By 1969, the war was at its bloodiest stage with the Federal forces sweeping the East and completely blockading the rebel enclave. Both sides desperately needed doctors and nurses and the few that remained were exhausted. In view of this, the Irish Red Cross was asked by the International Committee in Geneva to send medical personnel to Nigeria, but it was made clear that they would have to work on the federal side of the lines since Biafra as an entity was considered illegal by most countries.

I volunteered to go and within two weeks found myself on a plane to Lagos for the second time in my life. My first visit to Nigeria in 1960 had been to a country rising from its slumbers and beginning to flex its muscles. But *Pax Britannica* still ruled and you could travel safely all over the land. Then I was with my wife Doreen and our little daughter Mary and had spent a very happy eighteen months working as a doctor in University College Hospital, Ibadan.

My visit in 1969 was entirely different. This time it was to a country torn in two by war and one in which hatred and cruelty reigned supreme.

My motives in going were a combination of things. I felt it a duty, even a call, to offer my medical services, however small, to ease the appalling suffering I saw on TV. Certainly, neither money nor fame played any part in my motivation. Yet, also, if truth were told, there was a definite excitement about travelling to Africa again and in a special way about travelling to the West coast. I had fallen victim – like so many others – to the 'call of the coast'.

Ikeja airport – the major international airport of Lagos – was a hive of activity when I landed. Red Cross planes were being loaded with supplies from a large hanger with the international symbol of the Red Cross painted prominently on its roof and doors. Grey coloured military aircraft were lined up neatly outside the main terminal building and there was much coming and going of soldiers in khaki coloured jeeps.

It was steamy hot when I got off the plane and within moments my shirt was sticking to my back. But things had been arranged by Molly Murphy, that lady-like person who was the CEO of the Irish Red Cross at the time, and a car from the Irish Embassy was on the tarmac waiting for me. Almost before I could get my bearings, a pale thin young man approached and introduced himself by saying that he was from the Embassy and that he was instructed to bring me there as soon as I arrived.

I would stay there as our ambassador's guest until transport came for me. This was service indeed and I felt a great weight taken off my shoulders as we left by a VIP exit and weaved our way through the Lagos traffic which was, as ever, chaotic.

Eventually, we reached the embassy residence, a walled off compound in Victoria Island. Two honks on the horn and a smartly dressed gateman opened the sheet metal gate and we drove up to the front door. Our ambassador, Paul Keating, came out smiling and put me at ease immediately. He was a medium to low-sized paunchy, black-haired man with a sharp wit and a quizzical turn of his head – if you said something that either interested him or with which he disagreed. He greeted me warmly and led me into an air-conditioned study where books and papers littered occasional tables and where stacks of files spilled over on to any spare floor space. The pungent smell of a recently smoked cigar hung on the air and it was clear that Paul spent many an hour in this room perhaps reading, working, or just sitting

You could not ask for a more gracious host. That night we had a lovely dinner with wine and all the trimmings, and he regaled me with stories about his time in Nigeria. He was someone who enjoyed the good things of life, be it food or wine or literature or art or history. And as a raconteur, he was superb and had the ability to hold your interest in a serious subject and then in a flash have you doubled over in laughter as he recounted some funny or embarrassing incident from his ambassadorial life.

Afterwards I learned that he deplored the Irish missionary backing of the Igbos and blamed them, in particular the Holy Ghost Fathers, for prolonging the slaughter. Indeed, he worried that Nigerian-Irish relations might be permanently damaged.

Paul went on to the Court of St James a few years later but sadly died before he reached his 60th birthday.

I only had two days of enforced idleness and luxury in Lagos. A Red Cross convoy was due out before the weekend and I would get a ride with it to St Lukes Hospital, Anua, my final placement.

It took us two bone-jolting days to get there during which I suffered from continual dysentery. It was a journey that I prefer to forget. Yet when I did arrive at Anua, I suddenly felt fine, my stomach cramps disappeared and I was ready to work immediately. I told no one about my dysentery, for I feared that they might have sent me home!

CHAPTER 2

ANUA

St Luke's Hospital

I knew little of about St Luke's Hospital, more commonly called 'Anua hospital'.

At the time, it lay in the Eastern State of Nigeria, close to the thriving town of Uyo. It had been established in 1937 by Sr Mary Martin, the founder of the Medical Missionaries of Mary, the MMMs. It had grown steadily from a small dispensary and 'lying-in' unit to a bustling 280-bed hospital by 1969. It was then the flagship hospital for all Southern Nigeria.

Today Anua lies in Akwa Igbom State where the concept of Dakkada – a movement to energise people into self-belief – has spread to every area of public life, from health to farming to education. It is now a renowned teaching hospital and internationally respected. The acorn the young Mary Martin planted in 1937 has grown to a full oak tree.

Perhaps I was a little disappointed on my first glimpse of Anua hospital , for it was not a very imposing structure. Like many hospitals in Nigeria, it consisted of a central building facing the main gates, with two wings stretching forward, one on either side. There were several other low buildings on-site, housing individual departments and specialised clinics.

The nurses' home, as I remember, was between the left wing and a 2.0 metre high perimeter fence which completely enclosed the compound. The main entrance opened on to a tarmac road that led to the town of Uyo. There was a mission school across the road and some Kiltegan priests lived in a house nearby. My memory of the hospital layout is blurred not just because of the lapse of time but also because I have worked in so many places in Africa that I mix them up.

Two Memorable MMMs

Many MMMs – doctors, nurses, pharmacists and administrators – have served faithfully in Anua over the last 80 years, so it is somewhat invidious to highlight just two. But both had graduated with me in University College Dublin in 1957 and both were working in Anua when I arrived, so it is natural that I speak of them.

One was Ann Ward, a strong energetic fair-haired Donegal woman with a powerful personality and a compelling presence. Ann was an obstetrician with a special interest in vesico-vaginal fistula (VVF) for which she received many honours, including an Award of Merit from the International Federation of Obstetricians and Gynaecologists in 1997.

For those not familiar with the term VVF, let me explain that it is a condition in which there is an abnormal communication (a fistula) between the bladder and vagina. Consequently, the woman dribbles and smells of urine constantly. Sometimes the fistula extends to the rectum so that faecal incontinence occurs as well. It is almost always due to prolonged labour in which the pressure of the baby's head erodes the walls dividing these structures.

The sufferer is always isolated, rejected and ostracised *for life* by her husband and family because of the continual smell. Hardened as I am over the years to meeting people with all kinds of diseases, my eyes welled up with tears as recently as three years ago when I met a patient in Uganda with a VVF, in which cancer of the cervix had made operation impossible. I was glad to hear that she died in the arms of an African sister a few months later.

VVF still scourges women in the developing world. As recently as 2016, the MMMs reported that over 15,000 new cases occur annually in Nigeria.

I saw my first VVFs in Anua and assisted Ann in repairing them before she left for home. I never achieved her skill in operating on these cases but then few have. During the operations she chatted about her native Donegal, so like the highlands of Scotland, or would reminisce about the 'old days' and about her father who was a member of the first Dail Eireann – the first parliament in an independent Ireland.

In later life, I visited Ann in Drogheda where she was a semi-invalid, virtually bedridden. It seemed so unfair to see Ann, who had spent her life helping the sick, now reduced to relying on others for the most basic needs. Fittingly, Governor Udom Emmanuel, himself born in Anua, named the reconstructed gynaecology block after her in September 2015.

I had the honour of contributing to Ann's obituary in the *British Medical Journal* after her death in 2016.

Leonie McSweeney was the other sister doctor in Anua when I arrived. I hardly knew her during my college days but got to know her very well during my stay in Anua. Leonie was dark-haired, small and slim, and a diffident sort of person whose real personality one only saw when she smiled. Then her whole face lit up as the real Leonie shone through her dark eyes.

Both she and Ann were excellent surgeons; yet they were a complete contrast in other ways. Leonie was quiet, self-effacing and humble, whereas Ann was outgoing, a born leader and self-confident. Ann left her mark on the world stage; Leonie left it on the hearts of those she helped. She devoted much of her later life to helping married couples and was a recognised champion of the rights of the unborn.

After the war, Leonie moved to Ondo, also in Nigeria, where she promoted family life and natural family planning. She worked tirelessly at this and helped many a struggling couple by her understanding and compassion.

My Job in Anua

My job in Anua hospital was to replace Ann Ward and Jack Hickey. Jack was another Irish surgeon, who I was told had much experience in Adeoyo Hospital, Ibadan, many years earlier. He was a short-term volunteer with the Red Cross; in fact, he had volunteered before me. Unfortunately, he left before I arrived, so I did not get to know him at all. By all accounts, he was a meticulous surgeon. I would be hard pressed to keep up with either Ann or him. So it was obvious that I would have plenty of work to do, for within a few days, only two expatriate doctors remained: Leonie and myself. All the others had been evacuated home, either sick or exhausted. We had no junior doctors. Those had either fled or been conscripted into the army or had been murdered.

However, we had a third senior doctor, Ebom Etuk. Ebom was a Nigerian and, like most of the Nigerian doctors I met during the war, was grossly overworked and underpaid.

He was a good looking, tall, well-built, quiet and thoughtful man; although a superb clinician, I think that he was an academic at heart.

Ebom and I lived together in a house about 50 metre from a side gate that led to the hospital compound proper. Since the house was on a hill overlooking the hospital one had to descend, almost into a gully, when walking to work or answering emergency calls. This must have been a treacherous trip in the wet season when mud and water accumulated at the bottom of the gully, but in the dry season it was no problem.

During my stay, there were soldiers posted at all the gates of the hospital and by evening they were invariably tipsy from palm wine. Hence, both of us were afraid of night calls in case a drunken soldier would fire at us thinking that we were invading Biafrans. Although I was never shot at, I was accosted several times by a soldier waving his gun at me with an unsteady hand. In time I learned to shout well in advance that I was the doctor answering a hospital call. Happily this prevented any untoward accidents.

Since Ebom and I were on call every third night, we normally fell exhausted into bed on the free ones. As a result, we met but few times, even though we shared the same kitchen and dining room.

We had to do everything: paediatrics, surgery, medicine and – the most demanding – obstetrics, irrespective of whatever expertise we possessed.

I liked all these things and was a reasonable all-rounder, but Ebom – apart from being an expert surgeon – was totally passionate about a tropical disease called filariasis. Anua was an ideal place to study filariasis since two of its manifestations, *Calabar Swelling* and *Loa Loa*, were highly prevalent in the region. He taught me much about filariasis that was not in the textbooks and in doing so instilled in me a love of tropical medicine that I have never lost.

In quiet moments, he would be sad, almost downcast. I believe now that the war had affected him more than I ever suspected. Yet he never confided anything personal to me and I never asked. I really liked Ebom.

CHAPTER 3

MIRACLES, MAGIC AND MISTAKES

Mrs Joe Goes Fishing

Although my work in Anua was long and tiring and often frustrating for lack of facilities, it was really no different from that in any busy mission hospital. However, there were one or two incidents which I will never forget and which are worth recording. The first concerns a fish, a patient and me. I tell it as it happened

It was about 7 p.m. on the evening of 15 February 1969. It was still the dry season and I was tired after a long day. However, a man with a strangulated hernia had just arrived and needed urgent surgery, so I had no option but to operate on him immediately.

Our theatre – operating room – had two tables, side by side, so I got him placed on the one on the left and started by giving him a spinal anaesthetic. At this stage of my career, I was adept at giving 'spinals' and they were particularly easy to do in Anua, as the majority of the patients were very thin. I turned him on his left side and got him to bring his knees up towards his head so that he assumed a comma shape. The prominences of his lumbar vertebrae – we call them spines – stuck out like mountain peaks, and it was simple to insert a long thin needle between the appropriate ones to ensure anaesthesia from the umbilicus down. Once the injection had gone into his cerebro-spinal fluid, I rolled him over on his back and warned him not to sit up or even raise his head as a spinal anaesthetic can cause a precipitous fall in blood pressure. This is the cause of the very severe headache that we often see after a 'spinal'.

I scrubbed up in the usual way, draped the patient and made my incision in the groin area parallel to the left inguinal ligament. I was lucky in quickly finding the narrow orifice through which the hernia had squeezed itself out of the abdomen. It was clearly constricting the blood supply to the escaping bowel which was of a greyish black colour – the precursor of gangrene.

But luck was on my side. Within moments of relieving the constriction, the colour of the strangulated bowel changed to a greyish pink, and then to a solid pink, a sure sign that it was being revitalised. I pushed back the loop of intestine into the abdomen and was on the point of repairing the abdominal wall when I was interrupted by a hullaballoo at the door of the theatre.

There was much shouting, pounding and cries of 'emergency'. An orderly came running in gasping 'There is a woman outside … choking … Doctor….you must see her immediately… she go die….'

Such an interruption had never happened to me before, but the situation obviously demanded immediate attention, and so I replied, 'Let her in…let her in. …and put her…put her on the other table.'

He ran back and opened the door, and then five or six people rushed in carrying a lady who seemed quite unconscious.

'She's choking doctor….' 'Doctor … quick Doctor … Hurry….' Everyone was talking at the same time, but the essential message was clear enough.

'What happened? ... Did she swallow something?' I demanded, pretty alarmed at this stage.

'She swallowed a fish' they cried in unison.

'A fish? A fish? ... You mean a fish bone?

'No, No ... She swallowed a whole fish ... de fish be alive ... a live fish....'

This was a first for me.

Now I learned later that it is the custom – or certainly was the custom – for women to accompany their husbands when they went fishing on the banks of the local river. The women would chat happily while the men cast their rods. When a man caught a fish, he would turn towards his wife who would take it from the hook, put the fish – head first – into her mouth, and bite hard, severing the spinal cord. She would then throw the dead fish into a basket or calabash on the grass beside her.

Apparently my patient, Mrs Grace Joe, had been so engrossed in gossiping that she forgot to bite the head of the fish and instead had let it slither down her throat while it was still fully alive.

The fish got stuck there and the bulging pharynx now started to press on the structures around it, one of which – immediately in front – is the trachea or windpipe. Some air might get through depending on her position, the size of the fish and how impacted it was, but inevitably she would choke to death sooner or later, unless the fish escaped or slipped down into the stomach.

Grace's friends had carried her to a local hospital, but the doctor there promptly referred her to me.

And I don't blame him. She was *in extremis* when I saw her and I knew I had to take immediate action if I were to save her life.

I ignored all principles of hygiene, all ideas of anaesthesia, all elements of surgical training. I ignored the group of onlookers who crowded around me. It seemed as if the entire village had come at this stage. I called for an Allis forceps, a sort of tissue-holding forceps, and then got my assistant nurse to open the lady's mouth while someone else was told to hold the head steady. I looked in, depressed the tongue and then saw the tail fin of the fish waving up at me. It seemed as if the fish were still alive!

I applied the forceps gently and started to pull. All that happened was that the forceps came away in my hand with some bits of fish tail in its clasp. I asked for a second Allis and pushed both forceps down between the fish and the wall of the lady's gullet until I could grasp a decent chunk of the fish proper. I rotated the fish slowly while simultaneously pulling it carefully upwards. Suddenly, I had the whole fish.

Just as suddenly, a great cry came from the on-looking crowd. It was a real shout of triumph. More like the roar you hear when someone scores the winning goal at a football match. I cannot describe it. Within a few seconds, the woman sat bolt upright and, believe this --for it is true – she banged her head on the theatre light which was directly above her. It was becoming a comedy of errors for now her scalp was bleeding. However, I ignored this; I was too excited to bother about a small cut in her scalp. Indeed, I was completely caught up in the thrill of the moment.

I ran out of the theatre still holding the fish by the tail with the forceps, and I made for the convent to show my 'catch' to Leonie, who was off duty that night. I will never forget the look on her face when she saw my fish. She was sitting at table having her supper of sardines on toast. She told me later that although she was hungry, she could not eat supper after I left. Who can blame her?

When I came back to earth, I remembered my hernia patient. I found him fast asleep on the operating table and so I finished the operation in complete peace and ease. In its own way, the fact that Mrs Joe survived was a kind of a miracle although I suspect she had a headache for several days afterwards.

A Witch Doctor Refers a Case

Although I have had little personal dealing with witch doctors, they frequently referred cases to me. One case concerned a nineteen-year-old girl who came to my clinic in Anua with impending gangrene of the toes of both her feet. Her little toes were particularly affected, and when she came to me, they were cold, painful and turning black. I had never seen a case like this before and was at a loss as to its cause and as to what to do. One automatically thinks that a girl of this age may be pregnant and so I asked the obvious questions.

It gradually became clear that she was pregnant, but, because she was unmarried, she had gone to the witch doctor in order to procure an abortion.

He had put a spell on her lower abdomen, made a series of criss-cross cuts on her tummy and then given her an assortment of roots which, after boiling in water, she was instructed to strain and then drink. She did as she was told and repeated the 'medicine' every day for a week. On the eight day, she started to get pain in both her feet and this pain got worse and worse over the next few days. She returned to the witch doctor who wisely washed his hands of the whole affair. He took his money and sent her to our hospital with a small handwritten note asking the doctor on call 'to help this patient of his'.

It seemed clear that the root extract he gave had caused constriction of the blood vessels going to her toes. It was equally clear that I must somehow open up these vessels if I hoped to save her from losing her toes.

A more worrying development occurred shortly after admission. She now started to get pain in her fingers as well. These too were becoming cold and blue.

I have mentioned that, like all tropical surgeons, I was fairly adept at giving spinal anaesthetics. I knew too that one of the major effects of a 'spinal' is to dilate blood vessels by virtue of its knockout effect on the sympathetic nervous system. However, the effect of a spinal anaesthetic only lasts a few hours, and so it struck me that if I could give a continuous infusion of a spinal anaesthetic, it might allow continuous dilation of the constricted blood vessels. I had never done this before nor ever heard of it being done. But I was young and brash and went ahead anyway. In the event, we managed to keep the infusion going for 48 hours by which time her circulation was fully restored and she was pain free.

Nowadays one would consider giving a continuous epidural block in such a case, but I believe that this was a one-off case as far as a spinal anaesthetic was concerned.

My patient left hospital of her own accord and I never discovered whether or not she held on to her pregnancy, but I doubt it.

Luckily, I managed to bring some of the roots back to Ireland and got them analysed in Dublin, where I was told that they contained an alkaloid compound. Well-known alkaloids include strychnine, quinine, morphine and, significantly, ergotamine. Ergotamine causes constriction of blood vessels as well as contraction of the uterus.

So the witch doctor was using real 'medicine' after all, but in a completely reckless manner. Clearly, there was a method in his magic.

Juju, 'magic', was widespread throughout West Africa when I worked there. Spells, incantations, scarification, the use of roots and herbs and complicated rituals were handed down from generation to generation and were practised on a daily basis by witch doctors.

There was often a good scientific basis behind some of the medicines handed out, but 'bad' Juju was just as commonly practised as 'good' Juju. In 'bad Juju', the witch doctor would cast an evil spell on an enemy or on his cattle, and some witch doctors were uncannily accurate in the efficacy of their spells.

The Girl with the Goitre

As you can see, this is a personal account of my stay in Anua. I can give you no description of the countryside, no notion of the political situation and no accurate detail of how the war was fought. For these, you must go and search elsewhere.

But lest you think that all my medicines were successful, let me tell you of another case where I made a serious error, not in diagnosis or surgical treatment, but in a lapse of common sense.

A father and mother brought me a young girl of fifteen years of age who had a huge thyroid swelling. The swelling in her neck was unsightly and getting bigger. The parents complained that their daughter would never get married and that was a situation of the deepest concern to them. Such a tragedy could only be matched by having a barren wife.

They begged me to remove the swelling. I did not consider for long. If the swelling continued to enlarge, then soon the windpipe would be compressed and the child's life would be in immediate danger. Other things could happen too. Local nerves could be entrapped or she might end up unable to swallow. She might even go to a witch doctor who might 'operate' with dreadful consequences.

Besides, I reckoned that it is often easier to remove a large mobile growth than a small fixed one. So I agreed to operate.

I read the technique the night before in Farquharson's *Textbook of Operative Surgery* and re-read it early next morning. I would do a sub-total thyroidectomy, leaving enough thyroid behind so that she would not need hormone replacement for the rest of her life. As usual, in all MMM hospitals, the operating team prays for guidance and a good result before making the first incision.

I prayed harder than on other occasions and was rewarded with a relatively straightforward and bloodless operation. The little girl was brought back to the ward and had regained full consciousness before I finished my usual night round, about 9 p.m.

Next morning I discovered to my horror that she was dead. She had got a bout of coughing during the night, burst her stitches and bled to death. We had just one night nurse for 48 surgical patients in that ward and there was no way she could prevent this tragedy.

People think that surgeons just keep going on with the job as if nothing amiss had happened. But that is not true. Deep in our hearts, we grieve for the bereaved family, for the lost life, for the stupid careless mistake we have made and which we will not admit to anyone but ourselves. Surgeons are human, they make mistakes. Like other surgeons, I carry this burden to the grave.

I should *not have given in* to the parents. I should *not have operated* on this case in such poor conditions. I should *never have allowed* my patient to spend her postoperative time in a 48-bed ward with one nurse.

One good thing came out of this. I now warn my students to avoid making the same mistakes that I made. I hope they listen.

A Mission of Mercy?

In many ways, we were isolated from the actual fighting when I worked in Anua. The hospital served the local Ibibio population who, despite being sympathetic to the Igbo cause, did not suffer to the same extent at the hands of the advancing Federal armies. Nonetheless, Anua was close to the front line and, being situated in a slight valley with the Biafrans on one side and the Federal army on the other, we could hear intermittent mortar fire across the valley both day and night.

Federal soldiers 'guarded' the hospital compound, but we felt far from safe, and had there been a Biafran breakthrough, I am not sure how we would have managed.

Luckily, I was so busy working that I hardly had the time to feel fear.

However, I remember one incident – mostly due to my own stupidity – that caused me fear. I was told that Fr Tom Fitzgerald – a Kerry man – was very sick in a village about four miles away and needed a doctor. I immediately volunteered to go and see him. I suppose that part of this was to get away from the hospital for a few hours, but honestly I believe that my main concern was to aid a fellow countryman who was obviously in need of assistance. So I borrowed the hospital car – an old Land Rover – and threw in the few medicines we used all the time. These were chloroquin (for malaria), chloramphenicol (for typhoid), penicillin (for any infection), mebendazol (for worms), digoxin (for heart failure) and paracetamol (for fever).

I drove as per instructions and got safely to Tom who was not so sick after all but who had a clear case of lobar pneumonia. He lay on a kind of pallet in a local mud house and was tended day and night by kind and gentle local ladies. The place was pitch black inside, but, after a few minutes, my eyes grew accustomed to the darkness and objects became visible that I never thought were there in the first place.

The hut was spotlessly clean. There was a wooden table covered with a torn but clean plastic cloth. On the facing wall, a bowl of gaudy artificial flowers stood on a little shelf, above which was hung a picture of the Sacred Heart. You could be at home in rural Kerry and not notice the difference.

I left after giving instructions on how to inject the penicillin and, as I waved goodbye, I was very pleased with myself.

After the first mile on the road home, I heard a *thump thump* sound and wondered if the old Land Rover was going to conk out. I dreaded the idea of changing a tyre, partly because of the weight of the spare wheel and partly because I was uncertain whether or not I had a jack on board. Having a spare tyre or tyre-changing equipment or any object that can be stolen from inside or outside your car is an occupational hazard to this day in all developing countries. We have all learned this fact the hard way.

So you can see that I was concerned that I might be stuck on the road and left to walk two or three miles in the noonday sun before reaching Anua. And added to that I would have to leave the Land Rover stranded on the side of the road, a lovely picking for the numerous bands of thieves and bandits who scourged the area in search of loot. But then, looking at the road ahead, I suddenly saw spouts of laterite spluttering up into the air for no apparent reason.

At last, the penny dropped. It dawned on me that someone was raking the road ahead with gunfire, but I had no idea if it was the Biafran or Federal soldiers that were firing. I had obviously crossed the front line when going to visit Fr Tom and since they missed me on the way out, they would surely not miss me coming back. This was no joke. This was serious. I had no time to think rationally. I put my foot down on the accelerator and made that old Land Rover fly as she had never done before. We raced ahead until the shooting stopped.

I was in a cold sweat by the time I arrived at the hospital where I was greeted by laughing soldiers waving their machine pistols around carelessly and grinning broadly at my haggard face. For all that, they treated me with far more respect from then on.

I slept soundly that night, scarcely realising the danger I had been in. Such is the arrogance and invincibility of youth.

A Village Is Strafed

Apart from the incident coming home from treating Fr Tom Fitzgerald, I had only one other run-in with the fighting. For some reason, I was in the Land Rover again, driving through a village. Suddenly, I saw people running in every direction, men, women, and children, many carrying *peckins* (little children) on their backs. Bicycles were discarded on the road and their riders dashed off into the nearest open door. Children were running in all directions accompanied by dogs and cats, which seemed as bewildered as the humans. You could sense the terror as they scampered away.

This all happened in a moment, and then I became conscious of the roar of an aeroplane overhead. It was obvious that the village was being attacked and the main street was being strafed. I veered sharply left and brought the Land Rover to a jolting stop in a small lane that ran between the gable ends of two houses.

The attacker was a solo jet fighter flying in low over the village. He was firing his guns indiscriminately as he swooped down like a giant vulture. I could now see the pilot's face as he returned from the opposite direction to make another run at us. He seemed to be enjoying himself.

Time stood still as he came in again for a second swoop. It was like a scene from a film set, unreal, phony. Like as if it was not happening at all, just an illusion. And then he was gone. People crept out from their hiding places. Life resumed again. There was some moaning and sobbing, but no one was really hurt.

Obviously, this was all a mistake.

The plane was one of the zero jets, flown by Egyptian pilots, which the Federal Government brought in to strafe Biafran positions. Certainly, many of these pilots were unfamiliar with the local geography, for I am sure this village was in Federal hands at the time of the attack.

Ben's Toothache

I had much admiration for the sisters and priests who stuck steadfastly to their posts and their people throughout the war.

I know the Holy Ghost Fathers were deeply involved with the core Igbo people in the east, while the Kiltegan Fathers were just as involved with the Ibibio who lived slightly further towards the west. The MMM sisters and the Kiltegan priests were especially strong where I worked in Anua, and I developed a great and abiding friendship with many of them.

Naturally, I tended any sister or priest who got sick, and it did not take long to make me fairly expert in treating common tropical diseases such as malaria and dysentery. However, dentistry was another thing altogether, and I need not tell you that my knowledge of dentistry at the time was minimal.

There was one particular Kiltegan priest, Fr Ben Hughes, from County Longford, who approached me one day with a terrible toothache, and when I looked into his mouth, there was indeed a back tooth that looked rotten, smelled rotten and was exquisitely painful to touch. The nearest MMM dentist, an American sister, Jean Claire, was in Ibadan several hundred miles away and there was no dentist – that we knew of – anywhere locally.

Ben was a grand fellow, jovial, kind and strikingly normal, a latter day Falstaff. He was the sort of person you could sit beside on a long car journey without feeling awkward or uneasy in any way. But there was nothing jovial about him when I made him open his mouth and tapped his painful tooth with a cold steel forceps.

I knew straight away that the tooth had to come out, there and then, and that the journey to Ibadan was out of the question.

I told him that the tooth had to come out, a decision he took lightly. Indeed, I was embarrassed by his obvious belief that the young Irish doctor would do the job quickly and painlessly. After all, to the layman, pulling out a tooth would be child's play for a qualified surgeon.

So, early one Friday morning, Ben and I made our way to the 'dental suite'. This was located in an annex to the main hospital and housed a dental chair and dental instruments but no dentist. I felt quite confident as the two of us trooped passed the long queues of people who had gathered during the night to get food or treatment in the outpatient departments.

The Extraction

Having got Ben in the dentist's chair and injected local anaesthetic according to the instructions in *Dental Practices in the Third World,* I grasped the neck of the tooth with an instrument that looked like a pliers. Not a budge. I pressed down towards the roots but this caused pain. I then rocked the tooth gently from side to side as if I were extracting a difficult cork from a wine bottle. Not a budge.

I took a breather and started to separate the gum from the tooth all the way around so as to loosen it a bit. Sweat poured from my patient's forehead, saliva obscured my view of his mouth and now I too began to sweat, with big droplets splashing on my patients face. Yuk!

I had no suction, no mouthwash, no cotton buds, nothing. But I knew that I must not fail. So I kept at it.

I kept talking all the time about trivia in the vain hope of distracting him from his growing distress and my obvious inadequacy. I kept thinking of the famous story told of a Captain in the Royal Navy years ago when he 'engaged a rating in polite conversation thereby taking the rating's mind off the fact that he was inserting a red hot poker up his backside in order to cure piles.'

So, although Ben's contribution was muffled and infrequent, I knew that I had to keep talking. Dentists have the most captive audiences in the world. Even the President of the United States has to shut up when in the dentist's chair. But this could not go on forever.

Suddenly, a thought struck me. It was quite inspired, I reckoned afterwards.

I had kept a bottle of duty-free Irish whiskey in a drawer somewhere in this room. I intended to give it as a present to the Sisters before departing for home. I rummaged around and found the bottle.

'Drink this' I said '… it will help your pain and make you feel better.'

He obeyed like a lamb. I gave him a big slug. We had no glass, no cup and no drinking utensil of any kind. When he handed the bottle back, I downed a mighty slug myself.

It felt good and I felt stronger. I made one last effort to get that bloody tooth out. I wriggled it, pushed it and twisted it – all at the same time – hoping that I would not break his mandible. Ben seemed in half a daze whether from the whiskey, the floods of Novocain I had injected, or merely from fear, I do not know which.

At length, the tooth came out. Amazingly the roots were intact. I presented my trophy to Ben who pushed it away as if it were something evil. I was both relieved and proud and innocently excited.

'That was a tough one', I said casually despite a slight quiver in my voice. 'No bother to you Doc' came the reply 'But have you any aspirin? I have a terrible headache.'

So had I.

Going Home

I had a scare of a different sort at the end of my tour of duty in Anua. This time it was unrelated to guns, or shooting or MIG fighters or teeth. It occurred on my last day in Anua.

All departing personnel left by a helicopter, as the roads were unsafe. So, when the time came for me to leave, a helicopter arrived and I scrambled aboard happy and excited. Helicopters are noisy uncomfortable things but that did not dampen my enthusiasm. Yet as we rose in the air and I looked down on so many upturned faces and so many hands waving me goodbye, I felt a pang of sadness at leaving all these people behind, people I would never meet again, people that were now friends not just acquaintances. Leonie told me afterwards that when I had gone, the staff missed the smell of my old pipe almost as much as they missed me! I don't know if that was an insult or a compliment. I took it as the latter.

As soon as Anua and its nurses, doctors, patients and soldiers disappeared from view, we set our course to Port Harcourt where a Red Cross DC-3 was waiting to take a group of expats to Lagos.

As it happened, I was the last passenger to board the big plane and got several hostile stares from those already aboard who had been kept waiting for my helicopter to arrive.

But that did not bother me. Nor did it bother me that this was an ageing stripped down aeroplane in which we all sat facing each other on long improvised benches separated by a wide centre aisle. I sat contentedly with the others and breathed a sigh of relief as we soared up into the blue cloudless sky.

The DC-3 was a great old plane. It might have been a bit cumbersome and slow, but it was steadfast, reliable and always arrived safely at its destination. However, maintenance was poor during the Biafran War and even planes used by the International Red Cross were not always properly serviced. About twenty minutes from Lagos, there was sudden lurch and the plane tilted sharply to the right. And now those of us on that side clearly saw a large metal object sail serenely down to earth. It seemed to fall off the left wing. Only a few of us saw it and we were too stunned to utter a word. Was it an engine? It looked a big thing and yet was it possible for an engine to simply fall off a plane? No, not possible – unless of course someone had failed to tighten the retaining screws properly.

The pilot – whoever he was – righted the list fairly quickly so that, despite the plane plunging downwards for a few moments, we straightened up and continued our descent into Lagos as if nothing had happened. A crackling came over the tannoy, 'Don't worry folks ... that was an airpocket we entered just now ... No need for alarm ... stay seated.'

I never catch what they are announcing first time over the speakers in the airport, but I definitely heard the pilot reassuring us that time.

Nobody panicked. None of us went into hysterics, or shouted, or prayed aloud or cursed. We all stayed still and, quite unreasonably, assumed that there was no real danger, although something had definitely fallen off the plane or from the sky near us. Does that make sense?

We made a bumpy but safe landing and no one spoke much until after we disembarked. However, we all looked carefully at the wings of the plane and saw nothing amiss.

One big fat guy, who also saw something falling from the plane,muttered something about unidentified flying objects. Another guy said that we had seen a small flying saucer. Someone else remarked that it had been an optical illusion and went into all kinds of scientific explanations. No one listened to him.

I didn't care. I was in Lagos at last and would soon be home.

CHAPTER 4

1969: MILE 4 HOSPITAL

The War Goes On

Home was both a lift-up and a let-down. It was wonderful to be back to Doreen and the children. Only those who have been separated can fully appreciate the happiness there is in being reunited with those you love. Indeed, you only appreciate something when you lose it, and what can be more precious than re-connecting with the people you hold most dear.

On the other hand, you find that nobody is really interested in your story. They will listen politely for a short while but then a glaze comes over their eyes and it is clear that they are not really listening. Everyone knows that the quickest way to bore people is to invite them to your house for an evening and then subject them to endless pictures of your latest holiday. It was rather like that when I came home.

Consequently, I talked little about my experiences and tried to resume life as normal. Indeed, there were those who assumed that I had gone abroad to make pots of money and, worse still, those who told my wife that I was a bad husband to have left her and the children for so long. Furthermore, I was pretty certain that I had hindered any advancement in my career in Ireland.

But these things did not stop me volunteering to go overseas again and always I did so with the full support of Doreen who believed that it was the right thing to do even though it left her to mind the house and the children all the time hoping that I would come home safely.

So a short while after my return to Ireland, I was off again with the Red Cross, this time to work in 'Mile 4', another MMM hospital, so called because it was four miles from the nearest town, Abakaliki. It was, like Anua, in the Eastern Region and had recently been 'liberated' by the Federal army. I would be the only doctor there.

Mile 4 Hospital

The road to Abakaliki divided the hospital compound into two. The main buildings lay on the west side of the road. These formed a square with administration taking up one side, general clinics and outpatient clinics another, inpatient clinics the third and the operating theatres and obstetric wards the fourth side.

The sisters lived in a separate building, partly screened by trees from the hospital. There were two separate entrances from the Abakaliki road, one for the hospital and the other for the convent.

The doctor's house hardly warranted such a name. It was a small separate building situated midway between the convent and hospital with easy access to both. All you could see from the outside was a glorified hut with a door and two windows, well one and a half windows. The half one was high up and gave light to the 'bathroom'. The larger one was in the living room. This room served almost all functions: eating, sleeping, reading and entertaining! A small bathroom, cut out from one corner, was fitted with a washbasin and a long-drop toilet (deep-hole toilet). This had recently been improved with the provision of a seat and it was perfectly adequate for one's needs.

A bucket, filled daily with water by a fragile-looking housemaid, stood nearby and from time to time she or I poured lime down the hole. The lime killed most of the flies, insects and cockroaches that would otherwise swarm about and make life most unpleasant. We were careful with water. Water – except in the rainy season – was always a precious commodity.

Taking a shower was an art in itself. You had to use an overhead bucket and tip it over yourself once you had got a lather up. The timing was crucial. Tip the bucket too early and you are finished before you have washed at all. Tip the bucket too late and you are left with too much lather on your skin. Too little water in the bucket and you may as well not have bothered taking a shower. Too much and you regret seeing so much unused water going down the drain.

I always seemed to tip the bucket at the wrong time, either too early or too late, so that when I was finished, there was invariably some shampoo left in my hair, or soap in my eyes or lather on my skin.

The water felt cold. Many people enjoyed the tingling sensation of cold water on the skin. They are the lucky ones. I never got used to that.

The little house was perfect for me. I was near the hospital for work and near the convent for food. Besides, I spent hardly any time in my house, apart from sleeping there at night. This was because I worked all day, every day and took my meals with the sisters in the convent.

Before going to bed, I might read a little or write home by a bush lamp. These were precious moments when I could enter my own private world, cut out the bustle and babble of hospital life, and transport myself to a realm of serenity and peace.

My little house soon became my private Shangri La.

My First Attack of 'Fever'

I vividly recall spending three troubled days in my Shangri La when I got my first attack of fever – malaria. I had been doing a 'list' in the operating room since early morning when I suddenly felt dizzy. I was so dizzy that I rushed the end of an operation and hastily left the theatre saying that I would be back in an hour to do the next case.

I went to my house, took paracetamol and chloroquine and lay down. I now started to get a pounding headache and my shirt became soaked in sweat, which I put down to the effect of the paracetamol. However, within the hour, I was back on my feet and went over to the theatre again to finish the list. I had three more cases to do, and I lay down between each of them.

Eventually, I was finished and managed to make it back to my bed where I started to shake uncontrollably. I felt cold, freezing cold, although I had covered myself with two blankets and my travelling overcoat. I was thoroughly miserable as I lay there curled up, drenched in sweat, my head throbbing, my whole body shaking in a series of uncontrollable rigors, and a searing pain in my eyes whenever I opened them to the light – photophobia. This was cerebral malaria, brain fever.

I have little recollection of the next two days apart from having vivid dreams and being drenched in sweat. The sisters and the theatre staff minded me day and night, and by the third day, I was very much better, able to eat a bit and ready for work again.

I was to get many attacks of malaria afterwards but never as severe as that first one. I probably would have died had I not been so well minded. Our hospital was infested with mosquitoes and I am sure that the number of malaria transmitting bites we received far exceeded any protection afforded by our daily paludrine tablet.

My first attack of malaria gave me a huge respect for the disease and brought home to me the very real danger of death which that tiny organism, *Plasmodium falciparum*, poses. One advantage of getting and surviving a bad initial attack is that partial immunity is induced and so further attacks are far less severe.

Other, mostly milder types of malaria, hide in the liver once the first attack is over. We call the hiding forms *hypnozoites*. These *hypnozoites* can emerge from the liver from time to time over the succeeding years to give recurrent bouts of malaria. This type is typical of the India and has been stereotyped often by writers when describing recurrent attacks of fever in retired colonials.

I was to suffer from recurrent malaria in later life too, and these sicknesses, which occurred when I was in Ireland, puzzled me at first, until I treated them with anti-malarial drugs.

Our Holiday Home

On the other side of the road, right across from the hospital and compound, there was a narrow grass path leading to our leper colony. A small bungalow, like a gatehouse, stood just to the right of the entrance to this path. The little bungalow was to prove a blessing for us during these hard days.

Every weekend one of us – and by us I mean the sisters and me – would move into the bungalow and enjoy solitude, quietness and peace from Friday evening until Monday morning. I only got there once during my first three months, and that was because I was the sole doctor in the hospital and could never get time off unless there was a visiting doctor willing to do my work. Such visitors were rare. Any doctor who did come, for example that great missionary, Godfrey Hinds, were themselves exhausted and needed to rest.

However, an MMM doctor – Deirdre Twomey – came one weekend and generously allowed me to take a break 'across the road'. Deirdre – who had graduated with me – had worked in the hospital in nearby Afikpo for many years and was tired herself. Nonetheless, I accepted her offer with alacrity. I was actually excited at the prospect of real time off. I prepared for my 'holiday' by raiding the larder and taking enough eggs, tinned beans, bread and apple juice to last me for three days. We seemingly had an endless supply of apple juice, donated by some international organisation. We drank it morning, noon and night, so much so that I cannot now look at a bottle of apple juice without feeling nauseous. I had a similar turn-off from avocado some years later when working in Rwanda. Avocados grow everywhere in Rwanda.

So off I went on my holiday with a brown paper bag and small blue hold-all containing everything I needed for the weekend.

And now I cannot recall one thing about that weekend. Perhaps I slept for 72 hours!

The Lepers

The leprosy settlement was down the path from our holiday home. I would visit the lepers about twice a week and only see them otherwise if someone got suddenly ill.

I looked forward to my visits. The path to the lepers' huts ran through a marsh, which was alive with flying insects, cicadas, frogs, snakes and every sort of creepy crawly you can imagine. I loved to walk along this path just after dusk, when it was lit by a big blob of a moon sitting in a purple sky studded with a myriad of stars.

I used to think of Napoleon's remark to his generals when they emerged from his tent one night during the desert campaign in Egypt. They had been discussing the perennial topic of 'Is there a God?' and had come to the usual conclusion that God is a myth created by man.

Napoleon suddenly stopped and pointed up to the star-lit night sky saying 'Well gentlemen, how then do you explain all that?'

Like Napoleon, I used to feel very small and insignificant during these evening walks and like Napoleon I could only conclude that something bigger and cleverer than man was responsible for the order and beauty of creation.

It is strange, but true, that I have seldom, if ever, felt more tranquil and peaceful than during those visits to the lepers.

They were always delighted to see someone from the outside world. You could sense it in their welcome and see it in their happy faces. Visiting the lepers soon became a pleasure rather than a chore, and I know that I was not the only one who felt this way, for several others told me that they experienced the same thing.

The residents of our leprosarium were mostly long-term lepers with quiescent or burnt-out disease. Many had distorted faces, lacked ears or noses or had the classical 'leonine facies' with thickened eyebrows, broadened misshapen stubs of noses and coarse, blotchy skin. All had deformities of the hands or feet with missing fingers and toes. The loss of sensation that leprosy causes resulted in many scars from unrecognised burns and unnoticed trauma. Recurrent ulceration and infection of the skin required constant attention, dressing changes and meticulous hygiene.

There were children there too. Some had even been born in the leper colony. Sr Patricia O'Kane, from Belfast, taught the children the elements of the three 'Rs' (reading , riting, rithmatic) but they much preferred to draw pictures with crayons

and were surprisingly good artists. Patricia was a wiry bespecta-
cled woman with a kind heart who always offered to help people
– whether it was needed or not. She truly loved her lepers and
tried hard to teach the children but with limited success.

Patricia's interest in children did not stop with teaching.
She managed to pick up a number of orphans who were often
naked and always malnourished. I don't know where she got
them from, but she accumulated about twelve such stragglers
and housed them in a makeshift place off the pathway to the
leper colony.

The faith of the lepers was truly impressive. They had built
a little chapel and somehow got hold of a statue of the Virgin
Mary. I often stood at the entrance listening to a leper talking
to the statue as if it were an actual person. You may say this
is idolatry or superstition. But I have no doubt at all that the
real Virgin Mary listened and smiled and remembered these
conversations ahead of all the magnificent homages that are
given to her in places such as Lourdes and Fatima.

When I came home, I asked the medical students I taught
in Galway to collect money so that we could employ workmen
to improve conditions in the lepers' huts and buy toys for the
children and buy food for Sr Patricia's Kwashiorkor Unit.

They responded generously. And several pledged that they
would give up their 'beer money' for a month in order to help.
This is my chance to thank them publicly.

A Special 'Thank You'

There are many ways in which we can express our thanks when
someone is leaving. We can have a party, make speeches, give a
presentation, give fancy cards, write letters or we can hug and
embrace those who are leaving and tell them how much we
will miss them.

I still treasure the little things that I have received down the years, all trivial in themselves, but all important to me, and not the least, is the stringed collection of coconut shells the lepers gave me about a month before I left Mile 4. It is worthless in itself but beyond price in my eyes.

The Operating Theatre: The Heart of the Hospital

The operating theatre in Mile 4 was a simple square room off which there opened three smaller side rooms. One of these was for 'minor' cases and contained nothing more than a metal couch and a wooden table on which there were a few basic instruments. In the corner stood a mottled white washbasin for handwashing – when there was any water. It was the MMM custom to press the serrated rim of the metal cap of a bottle (usually the cap of a beer bottle) into a bar of soap, which could then be kept in place by a small magnet screwed to the wall. This conserved the soap and prevented it dripping all over the place. It is a custom I have used at home despite my wife's objections!

The second side room was a bit larger and combined the functions of a sluice room and a sterilising room for instruments, theatre gowns and drapes. There was a long table in the centre on which nurses re-powdered used gloves and straightened out crooked needles before washing and sterilising them for further use.

Lastly, there was the tearoom where we congregated for tea and dry biscuits between cases. This room was sparsely furnished with a few chairs and a low central table on which were a few books and a few dubious looking mugs. We changed into our 'greens' in a little annex off this room and scrubbed up there before entering the main theatre.

The focal point of the main theatre (operating room or OR as the Americans say) was the single operating table in the centre. By today's standard, it was primitive. There was a foot pump by which you raised or lowered the table, and there was a side wheel by which you could tilt the patient's head or feet in an upward or downward direction. This wheel was a nuisance since if you bent forward over the patient while operating, it stuck into your stomach, a most unpleasant feeling.

Overhead we had a good strong lamp, which we could manipulate to spotlight the 'operating field'. When the generator failed – as it frequently did – we had bright bush lamps to hand that also worked admirably.

An Epstein-Macintosh-Oxford Ether Vaporiser (EMO machine) stood at the head of the table. The anaesthetist, originally an unskilled orderly, was proficient in its use having learned the trade elsewhere. If required, he could intubate a patient, which proved to be life-saving on several occasions. Mostly, however, we worked with spinal anaesthesia, which the surgeon administered to the patient just before scrubbing up.

It was our custom to pray for the success of each operation just before we made the first incision. We prayed for everyone on whom we operated irrespective of tribe, creed, colour, wealth or occupation. This was a moment of quietness that was important for all of us. It was a sudden stop in an otherwise constant babble of conversation and noise that would go on as nurses came in and out, doors banged, instruments clattered on the table, and things were dropped on the floor. The brief silence was broken only by the sounds of everyday life that filtered in through the open windows. The outside world seemed very remote at such times.

For me, the theatre was a magic place. Once scrubbed up, you were insulated from the world. There was no telephone, no bleep, no scribbling on charts, but just you, the patient and your assistants. We became one little family helping one another and concentrating on doing our best for the person who lay at our mercy. I have had the most stressful moments of my life in theatre, but these have been as nothing compared to the genuinely happy times I have spent there. Of course, you get tired, even exhausted, towards the end of a long theatre session. But it is a peaceful tiredness. Call it the tiredness of accomplishment, of a job well done, of knowing you did your best.

Night Rounds

In the evening, after the bustle of operating all day, after the stars have come out and dark shadows lengthen, I always do a round of the wards and check every case that was operated on that day.

Hospitals are different places at night time. Gone is the hustle and bustle of the day. You enter quiet wards where many patients are already asleep and look peaceful and serene as they lie in the stillness. Here and there sad, happy, bright or wearied eyes will look up at you and you will exchange a smile or give a warm squeeze to an outstretched hand. The nurse will pad up quietly and whisper details about each patient. You pause at the very ill, adjust an IV (we make our own IV fluids) and above all ensure that no one is in unnecessary pain.

I am not exceptional. I believe that is how most of us feel who choose medicine as a life vocation. Frankly, I feel that it is an unearned privilege to be allowed to access the sick and destitute.

Nurses are in a better position to do this than doctors and I recognised this fact very shortly after I qualified. The intimacy that can be achieved between a patient and a nurse is akin to the intimacy between a mother and a child. It is hard to find a more wonderful and more fulfilling profession than nursing.

Triumph and Tragedy: A Post-Mortem Section

I am of course completely wrong if I have given the impression that all my theatre days were happy and successful. I was not always successful in what I did, I was not always happy at the end of the day and I was not always right when making a diagnosis or when choosing a particular surgical option. You will find plenty of examples of failure as well as of success in this book, but I hasten to add that, while this applies to all walks of life, it has a particular resonance with doctors, and especially with surgeons.

The following incident illustrates well the thin line between success and failure.

I was in theatre one afternoon doing an operation, the nature of which I cannot recall now, when Mona Kelly, a volunteer nurse from Toronto, came bursting in the door in an obvious panic.

'Dom…there is a woman outside who has just died suddenly in the middle of labour.'

'Are you sure Mona?' This was not what I needed.

'Yes, yes … She just died I tell you. Come quickly please … Please hurry.'

I dropped everything and went out with Mona to see what this was all about. Sure enough, there was a thin lady, obviously dead, lying stark naked on a trolley outside the theatre door. I had no idea how she died, but dead she was. No heartbeat, no pulse, eyes staring to the sky. Somehow my eye caught the shadow of a ripple passing down the front of her distended abdomen. I don't believe that I consciously considered what I did next.

Instinctively, I turned to Mona and grabbed the scissors that was hanging from her belt. I should tell you that anyone who was lucky enough to have a scissors made sure that it was tied to some part of their clothes, for otherwise it would 'disappear' pretty quickly.

With one swipe, I dug the point of the scissors into the dead woman's skin just below her chest and sliced her tummy open, right down to the pubis. I saw the womb bulging, almost rising to meet me. I slit it open in a similar fashion completing everything in a few seconds.

Technically, this was a 'classical' Caesarean Section, and, in this case, it was made very easy because there was no bleeding and no pain for my 'patient'. I extracted the baby without any trouble, cut the cord and immediately started to clear the baby's airway so that I could do mouth-to-mouth on the little mite.

Imagine my excitement when the baby – a little girl – began to breathe and started to go pink. I was thinking that I would write this case up for the *British Medical Journal* and would talk about it at every opportunity in the future. I was really euphoric and perhaps my pride is understandable, for a live birth after a post-mortem section is a rarity.

We kept our little girl for about two weeks in the paediatric ward where she thrived 'on the bottle' and became the centre of attraction for everyone who visited the ward. I remember her being handed over to her father on discharge and that was that as far as I was concerned.

It must have been two or three weeks later when I asked the ward sister how 'my special baby' was doing. I had rather expected that the family would have come to thank me or that some sort of recognition would have been made for my 'strong

Western medicine. And frankly, I was not a little put out that I had to make enquiries about my miracle baby rather than being kept up to date on her progress by the nurses.

'Oh she is dead doctor', the ward sister replied, and she said this in a matter of fact way that seemed almost indifferent, if not even callous. I was stunned. I knew the baby was good and strong when she left the hospital. What could have happened? Was it diarrhoea? Was it meningitis? Was it tetanus? 'What on earth happened to her?' I asked.

'They left her out in the bush and refused to feed her', she replied flatly. She looked at me as if I should understand. 'Dr Dom', she paused, and then added as if explaining to a fool, 'Don't you know our ways Dr Dom. The family believes she was Satan's child because her mother died before she was born. That is the belief of these people.'

'Did you know this before she was discharged?' I was annoyed, so angry. All my great work coming to nothing. That's how small my mind was, how vainglorious a person I had become.

'Dr Dom, everyone knew it. We were surprised that you let her go home.'

Everyone did not know it, I did not know it. But then again I had not bothered to ask who would take care of the child when she went home. I had not ever tried to learn about local customs. I still had to realise that you couldn't practise in another culture without knowing that culture and respecting its values, however much they differed from yours.

From then on, I became more sensitive to local customs and local mores. For example, I quickly learnt that having twins was considered bad luck, and that such babies were usually killed at birth. This may have been for the pragmatic reason that harassed mothers with large families to feed had neither the time nor the means to look after them.

However, the practice of twin rejection is by no means universal in Africa. The Bakubu in the Democratic Republic of the Congo (DRC) honour twins and give them preferment throughout life and the Yoruba mourn the death of a twin to the extent that the mother may commission a wooden statuette representing the dead one – called an *Ibeji* – which she will wash, adorn and 'feed' and pass on to the surviving twin, who will perform the same ritual throughout his or her life.

In those days too, and before it became popular in the West, I learned that breast is best. Not only did bottle fed babies suffer more diarrhoea and chest infections but also, precisely in those families where good hygiene prevailed, bottle-feeding indirectly led to more pregnancies. This was because in such households the mothers became fertile again far more quickly than if they were breastfeeding. Lactation inhibits the release of eggs from the ovary, thus postponing pregnancy for as long as the breastfeeding lasts.

Follow Your Conscience

So I was growing up. Some years previously, while working in Anua, I had seen a sister doctor tying the tubes of a woman after doing a Caesarean Section on her. This had appalled me, as the Catholic Church expressly forbade sterilisation at that time.

The Sister explained to me, 'Dom, this lady has seven children already. This is her second section. Look at that thin uterine scar. She will go home to the bush and get pregnant in a month or so, and she will rupture her uterus when she goes into labour. She will probably die before she reaches hospital or even after reaching hospital. And then her children will have no mother and will be neglected by their father. I know this place. I cannot take such a high risk. I have to balance medical risk against armchair ethics.'

I remained quiet and thoughtful.

Symphysiotomy

Ah, that dreadful word. You probably know what a symphysiotomy is. In case you do not, let me explain. It is a quick procedure, done under local anaesthetic, in which you partially or completely cut through the ligaments of the symphysis pubis that is the joint that fastens both sides of the pelvis together at the front.

The well-known Dublin obstetrician John Cunningham ('Divine John' as he was called) recommended it for prolonged or obstructed labour. It superseded the operation of pubiotomy – where you actually sawed through the pubic bones – as previously practised by the Italians.

Symphysiotomy was used in countries where medical facilities were sparse, underdeveloped or non-existent. For me in the 1960s, it was an ideal procedure, fast non-traumatic and easy to do on a woman who came to hospital almost moribund, after days and days of obstructed labour.

Sometimes the cause was a small, misshaped narrowed pelvic outlet where the baby could never come out naturally. We call this disproportion between pelvis and baby. On other occasions, the baby could not exit the womb naturally because of its awkward lie. Such obstructions were commonest with a transverse lie, perhaps a face presentation, or a breech or a shoulder. Spontaneous delivery in such cases can be likened to trying to push a wardrobe sideways out a door.

I did a symphysiotomy only when there was no time or facilities for a Caesarean Section and when there was obvious maternal or foetal distress. I tried to avoid severing the binding ligaments completely, because if I could get the baby delivered without too much widening of the symphysis pubis then

I knew – instinctively – that the mother would make a quicker and more complete recovery.

I had another factor to consider as well. I knew that mothers would have many repeated pregnancies and by doing a symphysiotomy I expected to make the pelvic outlet more expandable, ensuring that future deliveries would be normal and that I might prevent rupture of the womb and maternal death should the lady in question have another prolonged labour. I also knew that most women in rural Nigeria preferred to have their babies at home and always considered a Caesarean Section to be an abnormal and unlucky way of giving birth.

So I had good reasons for doing a symphysiotomy where I felt it was indicated and I was happy that I saved many a life using this technique, neither did I see the long-term complications such as we have found in Ireland. I would never have done anything that might inflict the sort of problems on women that emerged in more recent times. But of course I did not know at the time, and clearly see that there is no place for the operation, where there are good medical facilities.

Wrong Decision

I certainly did one symphysiotomy that I should mention, which is not greatly to my credit.

I was called one evening about 10 p.m. to the labour ward to deliver a baby who was a breech presentation. The baby's buttocks were literally stuck in the birth canal and would not budge. The mother had come into hospital this way having had no success with the witch doctor.

I started by hooking my fingers around the baby's knees and slipping the legs down, which I did successfully. I then tried to rotate and flex the head by inserting a finger into the baby's mouth and gently pressing downwards and laterally.

I failed to budge the head at all. I might have tried straight forceps, but I could see no way to slipping them on without tearing the mother or damaging the baby or both. Yet I could not get the head delivered and I began to fear for the baby's life.

I did a quick symphysiotomy, but this gave me no success either. It was obvious now that the cord was twined many times around the infant's neck and I wrongly believed that, if I could uncoil the cord, I might get the baby out. So I cut the cord, having first asked the nurse to look at the clock and give me four minutes to complete the delivery.

Can you imagine how I felt?

We had bush lamps, but it was still hard to see clearly. Some instruments had already clattered off the table on to the ground – God help sterility – and I was sweating profusely with my heart racing and my fingers becoming clumsier than ever. The nurse called out the minutes, 'One ... two ... three ... no baby ... four ... five ... six ... no baby.' Now, no foetal heartbeat, now the mother absolutely exhausted, and now I insert my hand deeper and feel around the head which seems large, larger than normal.

Yes, I should have known. This baby had a hydrocephalus. A huge enlarged head that could never come out the birth canal naturally. And now the baby was dead. Indeed, maybe the baby was dead for some time; perhaps, we did not really hear the tiny heartbeat with our tin foetal stethoscopes. Perhaps, we had imagined we had heard it.

Now, I had a further dilemma. Further mutilation of the mother would be unthinkable. A Caesarean Section was not on. So I had to do my first craniotomy. That is a nice way of saying that I had to cut into the baby's head and decompress it. Then I had to reduce the size of the head by nibbling its contents out bit by bit until the mutilated infant would be expelled spontaneously.

The Psalmist says 'My sin is always before me.' So too, for a doctor, our mistakes are always before us. What might have been … P.S. the mother survived.

Four Mistakes on a Sunday Morning

It was a Sunday morning. Early. I have always loved the early morning, especially in the tropics. And Sunday mornings were the most special of the week as there were no clinics, no operating and no crowd hassling you as you went from ward to ward. There was just the soft fading darkness, the sweet smell of night gradually disappearing and the silent wraith like figures of early risers, shrouded in mist and wrapped in formless cloaks to keep out the early morning cold. It was a time I liked to walk quietly around the compound, past the sleeping 'watchmen' and past those who had no place else to bed down except under the branches of a tree.

The stillness of the past night would soon give way to the raucous bustle of another day and the dreamy moon would soon fade before the blazing glory of the rising sun. But this Sunday morning was different. There was no time to gaze on the miracle of the birth of another day.

Instead, I became acutely aware of a hullaballoo at the front gate, which quickly shattered my reverie. I could hear and then see a group of people arguing with the hospital gatekeeper and it was clear that they were half carrying half dragging a young man who was obviously in distress.

I hurried forward to investigate and they explained that the young man had not urinated for two days despite having been forced to drink gallons of water. The poor lad was writhing in pain and his bladder was distended like a balloon right up to his umbilicus. It was obvious that he had a stricture of the urethra, somewhere between the bladder neck and the tip of his penis.

In those days, there were just two common causes of a urethral stricture: gonorrhoea or schistosomiasis (a tropical disease). Gonorrhoea accounted for over 90 per cent of cases, but this boy was fifteen years old and, I was pretty sure, he had a schistosomal stricture.

But what matter the cause, he was in agony and needed immediate relief. I cannot imagine how he had got from his home in the bush to the hospital. His companions carried him to the outpatients and laid him on a couch. I hustled them out and they left reluctantly, probably wanting to wait and see what I would do.

I was young and inexperienced and quickly decided to empty his bladder by inserting a catheter via his penis. This was stupid but seemed logical at the time. So hardly had I cleared the room when I cleaned the tip of his penis, squeezed some xylocaine gel into its external opening, and then proceeded to insert a catheter through it up towards his bladder. This was painful. I had not allowed time for the anaesthetic to work. First mistake.

He had been writing and moaning in agony before, but now he screamed, I had tried a wide bore soft rubber catheter but it would not pass. I guessed that the stricture was probably one of many along the course of the urethra, a not uncommon finding in schistosomal disease. I tried a second catheter with the same result. Second mistake.

I then tried a straight hard plastic catheter and once more failed to get past the first stricture. Third mistake.

The boy's cries were pathetic and I was now suffering with him. As a last resort, I used a metal catheter but this time injected sodium amytal intravenously into a vein in his arm. Sodium amytal is a short acting barbiturate with a similar action to penthothal or propofal but far more dangerous. He went asleep instantly and, as he did so, I pushed the metal catheter firmly through the stricture and into the bladder so that the pent up urine poured out freely.

Thank God! He woke at this point and his relief was instantaneous.

Although I had abolished his pain and let the urine flow, I had now made my fourth mistake. The metal catheter had torn his urethra and blood began to seep out of his penis.

The next morning I partially redeemed myself by inserting a self-retaining balloon-tipped catheter into his bladder via his abdominal wall, we call this procedure a *suprapubic cystostomy*. This would short circuit the urethra and allow time for his torn urethra to heal. Finally I transferred him to Enugu where I knew they had far better facilities than we had.

The sad truth is that had I drained the bladder immediately via a *suprapubic cystostomy*, the boy would have had little or no pain, and his bladder would have come back to normal size within minutes. He could have had elective surgery on his strictures at a later date. Any surgeon knows that this is the correct thing to do.

I never found out the name of that boy. I hope that he did well afterwards. Who would want to be at the mercy of a young surgeon struggling alone, unsure and unsafe?

Mission versus State Hospitals

Mile 4 was a 'mission hospital'. Like other mission hospitals, it was accused of trying to convert patients to Christianity and criticized for charging for its services, whereas State hospitals were non-denominational and free of charge.

In answer to the first charge I can vouch for the fact that we never tried to convert any patient to Christianity and that we only discriminated on the basis of medical need, not on the basis of race, colour, gender or beliefs.

As regards charging a fee for services let me say that the charge was minimal and fell well below the economic rate and that we could only continue to provide a service because of a generous subsidy from the home country in the 'West'. People who were obviously indigent were treated free. Emergencies were treated immediately and were only charged if they could afford to pay. In addition, there is the universal truth that people only fully appreciate a thing or service if they pay for it or at least contribute towards its cost.

So why did people flock to mission hospitals when government ones were 'free'?

I believe that it was because they knew that care in Mission Hospitals was far better than anything found in the state-run ones.

In my own limited experience of state-run District Hospitals I was struck by the apathy of the staff, the dirt of the wards, the neglect of equipment and the general air of misery that prevailed among the patients.

When Fr Martin Downey brought me around the District Hospital in Chikwawa (Malawi) a few years later, I found things had not improved. Perhaps I was unlucky to visit at a bad time or unlucky in the choice of hospital I visited. I do not know.

But care was not the only problem that beset 'free' State hospitals. It seemed to me that there was far less overt corruption in mission hospitals. In State hospitals, one often had to pay the nurse for medicine, pay for an intravenous (IV) infusion and one always paid for a blood smear.

Connivance in corruption was also common. We frequently saw people who supposedly had an operation in the past – for which they had paid well – but in whom the surgeon had only made a skin incision. This was very common in cases of hernia and there is no doubt that scam surgery was practised widely in those days.

Staff Conditions

It is not really fair to castigate State hospitals as I have done without appreciating that working conditions for the staff were often so bad as to rob them of any initiative or reason to take pride in their work. Also salaries were not as high as in Mission Hospitals and sometimes salaries were not paid on time or not paid at all. Nor was the road to advancement as clear-cut as for their counterparts in Mission Hospitals.

Certainly, in my time, the government salaries paid to doctors in rural areas, of what we then called the Third World, were appallingly low. These doctors worked single handed seven days and seven nights a week and, although they became very skilled clinicians, they had no time for themselves, no money and no facilities for professional advancement.

Many had to work small farms as well as in order to live. They needed every penny they could earn because, as a doctor, as someone with a job, they were expected to support, feed and educate not only immediate family and relatives, but also those from their own village and their own tribe. While any relative could make free of their house, they were also bound to employ them as paid servants and generally share their 'wealth' with them.

Indeed, I knew Professor in Central Africa who worked in the hospital every morning, worked on a small plot of land every afternoon and wrote articles for renowned international medical journals in the evenings!

CHAPTER 5

FAITH OR FOOLISHNESS

'A Suspension of Disbelief' (Coleridge)

On 20 July 1969, the first men set foot on the moon. This was an historic event, a supreme triumph of science and a cause of general celebration throughout the world – apart from the Soviet Union whose space programme had failed to win the race with the United States.

But for me, working in the Mile 4 Hospital, the news of this achievement meant little. The Biafran War was still raging, people were dying of starvation on every side and atrocities were being reported daily. Facilities in Mile 4 and other hospitals were stretched to breaking point.

In the midst of so much suffering and death, the transience of life was an ever-present fact. And although we all know that life is a one-off business, we seldom take time to seriously think about what happens afterwards – if anything.

Working in Mile 4 forced me to think about such things and confirmed in me my conviction that life has no real purpose if death is the end of everything. Is that naïve? Wishful thinking? Stupid? Where is my proof?

Atheists and agnostics always demand proof. Incontrovertible proof.

It should be evidence based they say. Rational and logical.

This is not new thinking. Doubting Thomas would not accept anything at variance with human experience unless it was

'evidence based'. Indeed, Jesus himself talked about this generation as always 'seeking signs', before believing anything new or
out of the ordinary and, I have often made the point that if a
glorified Jesus Christ walked down Oxford Street or 5th Avenue
or appeared in Red Square today, we would not believe it.

Indeed, many of those who witnessed it would soon begin
to doubt themselves and be convinced, in time, that they had
been subject to mass hysteria or fooled by a clever con.

And so I tell the following story as I remember it, not
because it is inexplicable but because it is true.

The Prophet David

It was a constant source of irritation to me that almost every
day a group of white-robed men came into the hospital
compound making prayers and incantations over 'my' patients,
and impressing everyone with strange gyrations, as they raised
their hands to heaven invoking the gods of the sun and sky, to
grant patients' requests. I suspected, but could not prove, that
they were paid money for such services and this only incensed
and frustrated me the more.

Finally, I decided to approach the man who always led
them into our compound. He was somewhat taller than the
rest and, unlike the others, his headdress was embellished in
the centre with a bright red stone, perhaps a ruby. He was definitely a good-looking fellow, not much over 40 years old, and
had very dark piercing eyes that seemed to see through you.

I went up and accosted him one day, as he and his troop
were about to leave.

'Who are you... and what right do you have coming in
here to a Christian hospital.... with all your pagan carry-on?'

'I am the Prophet David', he replied gravely, 'and these are
my disciples'.

There was nothing amusing or silly in his answer. He was clearly genuine and certainly courteous. Indeed, his manner was altogether engaging and agreeable and he was far more calm and serene... than I.

'You are... upsetting my patients....' I stuttered, taken aback.

'I do not want to have you coming here. It is not right.'

'*Dokita*, do not worry. We only bring peace and blessings. Even the sisters do not object to our visits.'

I knew he was right. I had brought the matter up with the Sisters on a few occasions and they had laughed it off and told me not to worry, saying that this kind of thing was part of the local culture and that we should not let it upset us.

They pointed out rightly that Juju Hill was close by. Juju Hill was feared and revered by the locals and not a little feared by expatriates too. All kinds of stories about the going-on in Juju Hill circulated from human sacrifice to the enactment of strange esoteric rituals. Today I understand that it is part of the Abakaliki metropolis, itself the capital of the Ebonyi State.

But I was 'young and foolish' and Juju Hill meant nothing to me.

So it was with a clear mind and by design that I met up with the Prophet David a few days later. I knew that he generally came around noon.

This time there was no doubting our mutual animosity. I told him clearly.

'I am forbidding you from coming here again and expressly forbidding you from preaching your false gods.'

On this occasion, several of the ambulant patients had gathered around us and were intent on listening to everything we said.

Prophet David raised both his hands high like Moses of old. You could feel the intensity of his personality like a physical force.

'So you want to turn away our Gods ... perhaps you are afraid of them ... *Dokita*,' The last word was said with a sneer.

I was losing face and he sensed it. I could not think of a reply but just stood there like a fool.

'Are your Gods more powerful than mine?' he now demanded in a loud voice. So loud, in fact, that more and more people gathered around the two of us.

I fell into the trap.

'Of course my God is stronger' I replied, and then added unnecessarily 'He can do anything'

Prophet David must have smiled to himself. He had baited and trapped this arrogant white doctor, this know-all *mzungu*.

'Can he make it rain?' His voice carried a note of sarcasm and the definite quiver of a challenge.

'No problem.' I answered without even giving it a thought.

My arrogance or let us say my Faith was unshakeable, unassailable and utterly fearless.

'Well', we all looked up to the clear blue sky, 'Let it rain'. There was complete silence. Which I broke angrily.

'Tomorrow, tomorrow at noon, it will rain.'

I was defiant and definite. He smiled gently and swished away with his followers saying that they would come back on the morrow at precisely noon. I was left standing there alone, while the onlookers quietly slipped away to their various wards and to their various tasks.

At supper that night, I told my story to the sisters. They listened politely but, as far as I can remember, if I got any advice, it was *not to show up* at noon next day.

That night I prayed very hard. I mean very hard. Doubts came into my mind. Not about the ability of God to listen to me and make it rain, but because it began to dawn on me that my request was frivolous. Here I was in the midst of disease, poverty, starvation, war, rape, murder and every conceivable agony that humans can endure. And here I was asking for such a silly thing.

At length I fell asleep. So what, if it didn't rain, then that was the will of God and I would learn a lesson in humility. But still I was quietly confidant!

Next day dawned still, clear and cloudless. The sun rose and shone down on the dusty sandy hospital square. By ten to twelve, there was a gathering of patients and staff and onlookers from the surrounding village lined all four sides of the square. Some of the patients had their IVs with them. I can still see one pregnant lady, on a drip to induce labour, who got her family to roll her bed out so that she would get a good view.

But the centre of the square was empty. That is except for me. In my shorts, stethoscope around my neck, pen and notebook in the breast pocket of my short-sleeved shirt.

Nor was there a nun or priest in sight. But I did not care; this was between David and me.

Sure enough, at five minutes to twelve he arrived, followed by his entourage. He strode towards me and we greeted each other with a courteous African handshake in which we gripped each other's hands, then interlocked our thumbs and finally struck our breasts.

'The rain will come' I said solemnly.

He nodded and waited expectantly.

Overhead there were a few wisps of cloud, high up, not threatening. I grasped David's hand again and held it in mine so that both our palms faced up.

It was now noon. I closed my eyes and asked the Lord to do whatever he wanted.

A very gentle breeze, no more than a flicker, stirred the atmosphere.

And then both our palms were wet. The drops of water were clear and obvious, but you could not call this a shower of rain. It was more like dewfall.

The Prophet David stood transfixed for a moment or two. He bowed and graciously acknowledged that my God had stronger Juju than his, and then, with all the dignity or a king he left, followed silently by his disciples.

I almost pitied him.

No other comment was made, no other words said.

The crowd dispersed quietly. There was no clamour, no shouting and no alleluias!

I went back to work thankful but not surprised. After all, I had asked my Lord, who could do everything, to do a little thing for me and so 'He' had obliged.

Statistics show that it can rain on approximately five days each July in Abakaliki.

There are no statistics about the time of day or night it can rain. No statistics exist about the chances of rain on a particular day, at a particular time and in a particular place.

I have told this story several times but never written it down.

I vouch for its truth. There are those alive who can vouch for it, including the Prophet David. However, he never came to visit us again.

This story is either true or not true. Sometimes I doubt it myself and have to say 'Dom ... You were there ... c'mon you fool ... it really happened....'

CHAPTER 6

MILE 4 HOSPITAL AGAIN

Peace at Last

My second period in Mile 4 was in 1977. An uneasy peace prevailed. But people were rebuilding their lives and looking to the future not the past. Everyone was weary from the long years of war and famine and no one wanted to go back to those days. The hospital was also in rebuilding mode, but now that international funds were drying up we found it difficult to pay for medicines and equipment, not to mention salaries. Somehow, we managed by scrimping and saving and working long hours. But none of this could have happened without the wholehearted cooperation of the staff.

This time I went back with my eldest daughter Mary, then a dental student in Trinity College Dublin. Mary had been barely two years old when Doreen and I first went to Nigeria and was excited at the prospect of making a return visit to a country she could only remember from faded sepia photographs. I was excited too for I would relieve a sister doctor for three months and at the same time be able to share 'Africa' with a close family member and see first-hand how post-war Nigeria was progressing.

Mary – like most twenty year olds then and now – was full of vitality and the idealism of youth. She lived with the Sisters in their convent and they mothered her. Of course, they got all the stories and tales of 'goings-on' that only a young girl can bring, and she brought many, as she mixed with everyone, chatted to all and was very much in demand everywhere she went.

I lived in the same little bed-sit I had occupied during the war.

It was in my quarters that Mary found a gecko egg, which she carried home to Ireland carefully and which hatched in her hand in our kitchen. She let the tiny bewildered gecko free and to this day wonders how or if he survived in our harsh northern climate.

Mary often followed me on rounds, and it was here that she first saw leprosy, malaria, and TB and, of course, she also saw many mothers giving birth. Africa was a wonderful experience for her and she enjoyed every minute she spent there. It was also a wonderful thing for me as it cemented a father-daughter relationship that is more precious than gold.

Of course, there were some changes in personnel when we arrived. Sr Bernadette McConville, my previous boss, had been succeeded by Sr Carla Simmons, an American MMM. Carla was a sound practical person not afraid of work and not overly bound by unnecessary or trivial rules. All MMMs have specialised training and Carla was a trained social worker, but in time I discovered her secret desire to become a medical doctor, something that seemed an unattainable dream.

Some dreams do come true. When I returned to Ireland, I pleaded her case with Martin Newell, the President of University College Galway, to use his privileged position to have her admitted to pre-Med in Galway. He agreed and she eventually qualified with distinction as a doctor in Galway. I have met Dr Carla from time to time since, most recently in Uganda, where we rehashed old stories and shared experiences and laughed over trivialities we thought important in 'the old days'.

Otherwise the staff of Mile 4 Hospital was much the same, and I even recognised a few of the patients. At least one of them remembered me. I was sitting in the outpatient clinic one morning, faced by the usual long line of prospective patients, when the nurse ushered in a shrivelled little grandmother.

'You didn't leave us after all' she croaked. All the time she was sniffling and cleaning her dripping nose with her sleeve. 'I knew you wouldn't ... But you were a long time away on holidays.'

Seven years is a long time for a holiday.

She searched deep down in a pocket and produced a small piece of paper, folded many times and covered in grime.

When I unfolded it, I could see the writing was in my hand. 'Return to see me on Friday' followed by my scrawled signature.

'My appointment' she announced proudly. 'I came every month but you were never on seat.' She meant that I was not there.

The note was dated 9 April 1969. Could she have come here almost 350 times expecting to find me?

Now that was patient loyalty. As they say in Nigeria, 'that pass all'.

It was amazing how one picked up the thread of life after being away for so long. Within a few days, I was fully back to work as if I had never left.

Life was altogether much easier than it had been ten years previously. Nonetheless, there were still many shortages. Food and petrol were expensive and more and more hungry and sick people appeared at our hospital gates. My workload increased by the day, but I was young, strong and healthy and, most of all, I was happy to be of some help where there was so much need.

Hernia

There is no doubt that any doctor working in sub-Saharan Africa quickly becomes expert in operating on hernias. In those days having a hernia in Nigeria was as common as having acute appendicitis in the West. We generally attributed this to the fact that Africans carry heavy loads on their heads in contrast to Europeans and Asians who carry everything by hand or else drag their belongings in suitcases – a sure recipe for shoulder pain!

Undoubtedly, carrying loads on one's head confers a graceful stylish gait and prevents damage to shoulder joints. However, the price paid is an increased pressure on the spine, which transmits to the abdomen and forces segments of the intestine out through any weak spot in the abdominal wall. Since males have a potential route via the inguinal canal – a route that let the testes descend to the scrotum before birth – one can expect 'inguinal' hernia to be far more common in males than in females. And so it is.

At first, the person can squeeze back the contents of the groin swelling (scrotal swelling in a man) back into the abdominal cavity. These contents are normally a loop of intestine and perhaps some fat. This is called a reducible hernia. However, as time goes on the loop of intestine may twist on itself ('torsion') or become blocked or compromise its own blood supply at the narrow point where the intestine exits the abdominal cavity. This is an irreducible hernia.

The narrowing at the exit causes strangulation of the gut. At first, strangulation is reversible once the pressure is relieved, but in time becomes it irreversible, with consequent gangrene (death) of the trapped intestine. Bacteria escape through the gangrenous gut wall and infect the peritoneum – the protective membrane that covers the intestines. Peritonitis and subsequent death from septic shock become inevitable.

Hence the absolute necessity to operate on anyone with a strangulated hernia.

At least, three or four times a week, one would have to deal with strangulated cases, where the patients were very ill, vomiting and dehydrated. These patients were sure to die unless surgery was performed as soon as possible.

Filariasis

Filariasis was another cause of scrotal swelling. In this disease, a small tropical worm blocks the lymphatics which drain excess fluid away from different parts of the body. When filariasis blocks the lymphatics that drain the scrotum, the scrotum swells – often enormously – and sometimes to the extent that the sufferer may need a wheelbarrow to carry his affected organs. You can drain and tightly bandage these huge scrotal sacs as often as you like, but they quickly fill up again, leaving the patient worse off than when you first saw him.

When the worm blocks the lymphatics that drain a lower limb the result is a huge swollen leg ('elephant leg') for which modern day surgery can do little. When lymphatics from the upper limb are involved then the arm may swell to ten times its normal size.

In the West, huge swelling of an arm and hand can follow cancer of the breast or irradiation of the axillary glands. The modus operandi is the same as in filariasis – blocked lymphatics.

Chief Joseph's Scrotum

I have no idea what age Chief Joseph was when he came to visit me. He had a fine face, lovely ebony skin, firm eyes and a noble head covered with a mass of black hair going grey at the temples. He was the kind of person that you felt honoured to be with, and he exuded an air of serene authority that only comes with the wisdom of the elderly. He looked at me keenly and must have wondered what this young *mzungu* could do for him. But I suppose he was desperate and had nowhere else to go.

He told me that he was probably 50 years of age. Yes, that made him old enough. He then pulled up his jellaba and showed me his enormous scrotum. It was so big that you could not see the penis which was presumably buried somewhere in it vastness. This was filariasis, worse than I had ever seen before.

'You must operate on me doctor' he said 'and you must get rid of this curse'.

I was flummoxed. 'I do not think I can really help you much. If I operate, I will certainly take away your 'power', your manhood, and most likely you will end up dribbling piss all the time'

'I don't care.'

'But what about your wife ... I mean ... your wives?'

'I am not a man now. Because of this thing'

'And have you children? What will they say?'

'I have many children, about 20 or 30 I think. They want me to go to you'

I was afraid of operating on him. I knew it would be very difficult technically and that infection and bleeding would be almost inevitable. I had a 'gut' feeling that I should leave him alone. It was the nurse who persuaded me to change my mind.

'He cannot be buried under the ground like his ancestors if he dies with such a gross deformity. He will be left in the bush for the wild animals and his soul will wander around the land for evermore without finding rest'

We operated on this kindly 'old' man later in the week. I simply cut away everything and was lucky to have left him with fairly good control over his bladder.

Almost every bad complication that could occur did occur, including sepsis. But he lived, and walked out of the hospital a month later, grateful and happy. Minus everything. Yes, everything.

I saw him two months afterwards when he brought me a pair of chickens. I understand he died within the year and got a proper funeral and I am sure he rested in peace for evermore. I had learned something about native customs from Chief Joseph but had not learned enough, as other cases continued to teach me.

Time Off

On most afternoons when I was free, I would take a short walk past the back of the hospital, across a grassy patch, then over a little stream and finally sit myself on a warm stone in the shade of a tall tree surrounded by a thicket of dense bushes.

Here I was alone. I could doze, I could pray the rosary, I could, as the saying goes, 'sit and think, or just sit'. I used a stout stick to ward off snakes and frighten anything else that might be lurking in the bushes, and I would jump quickly over the stream to avoid the notorious Mango or Red fly (*Chrysops*) whose bite can inject the larvae of *Loa Loa* (the African eye worm) into unsuspecting humans.

Loa Loa is a feared manifestation of filariasis. It is a fascinating condition. Once the larvae mature they creep across the eye, just under the conjunctiva.

Here they are easily seen by another person and can be removed if snared before they disappear to deeper parts – which they will in a few hours. Such cases were common in

Mile 4, but when one appeared in an immigrant in Dublin a few years ago it was rare enough to warrant publication in a local medical journal.

The worms also love to move around under the skin where they cause lumps and bumps called *Calabar swellings.*

Visitors to West Africa react more angrily to the *chrysops* bite than locals who are immune to the condition because of exposure at an early age.

No wonder I was careful to avoid the breeding places of these flies.

However little did I know that I was under surveillance by humans rather than by flies during these walks. So imagine my surprise when, one afternoon, I found a clear path had been cut for me, right up to my special rock. Obviously someone with a macheté had done this job pitying the hopeless white man who went 'out in the midday sun… like a mad Englishman'.

Ever since then I know that you are never alone in Africa. Whenever or wherever you go there are eyes following you. They are there to protect you if you are a friend. But possibly there for less kind reasons if you are not.

The Daily Gatherings

Anyone who has worked in a hospital in rural Africa is familiar with the lines of people who gather before dawn at the gates, hoping that they and their children will get seen before the day is out.

In countries such as Zambia or Ethiopia these long queues are quiet and shadowy. The people who gather are quiet – almost wraithlike – and mostly covered in shawls or blankets to keep out the cold night mist. There is little talk, just a murmuring when the 'doctor' passes by.

On the other hand, in West Africa, in my experience, the waiting crowds are boisterous, noisy, and argumentative and have all the impatience of spoiled children. The noise reaches a crescendo when they see you entering the compound.

Mostly, however – again in my experience – the West African is happy-go-lucky, gay and full of ready-made laughter, even in the midst of grief and sickness. I hope that they never lose that spontaneous good humour which distinguishes them from the duller races of Northern climes.

Pay as You Go

As you approach the outpatient clinic in Mile 4, there is a large leafy tree. It stands on its own like a sentinel guarding the hospital. An old woman used to sit in its shade all day long from Monday to Saturday and we would see people casting the odd coin in her direction. The old hag was dressed in rags and refused to take any clothes the Sisters offered her. But she was not a nuisance, and we always made sure that she was given food and water every day for which she thanked us by calling down every god in heaven to bless us and our ancestors and to give us many strong children. Which made the celibate Sisters laugh!

I learned some years later that she was found dead under the tree one morning. I don't know who took the body away for burial but I do know that among the objects found beside her was a battered tin box full of pennies. Apparently she had been collecting a penny off each person who visited the outpatients over the years and had accumulated a small fortune in copper coins.

It's a strange world.

Today Abakaliki and 'Mile 4' are thriving modern places full of bright energetic people who live in peace and prosperity in a new Nigeria that has emerged from a cloudy past, has cast off the shackles of colonialism, and looks to the future with confidence and optimism.

For all my nostalgia, I would not wish it to go back to the 'good old days'.

CHAPTER 7

A NIGERIAN ROAD TRIP

African roads are littered with the burnt out, overturned wrecks of lorries, mammy wagons, *matatus* (in East Africa), buses and cars. To describe the carnage when a mammy wagon runs straight into an oncoming vehicle, or careers wildly off the road as it attempts to round a sharp bend, is to be lost for words.

But if you take a proper bus, say an Akamba line bus, from Kampala to Nairobi or from Blantyre to Lilongwe, then things are much better and accidents and breakdowns – though common – are fewer. Indeed I have enjoyed such trips and have always been lucky enough to sit beside a pleasant travelling companion.

However, I must now go on to describe one road journey in Africa that neither my daughter Mary nor I will ever forget.

As the time for going home from Mile 4 drew nearer our excitement mounted at the prospect of eating proper food, sleeping in clean sheets and of having water and electricity assured all the time. Most of all we longed to see everyone at home knowing that their excitement, like ours, must be mounting by the day.

Our plan was to drive to Ibadan and stay there before going to Lagos and taking the flight back to Ireland. I wanted to bring Mary to Ibadan and show her the house where she had lived with Doreen and me when she was a toddler. This meant a long road journey.

In Ibadan we would stay in Eleta with the MMMs. Sr Jean Claire, had agreed to let Mary help her in the dental clinic, so that was an added bonus. The MMMs ran St Mary's Hospital at Eleta, their first hospital in Ibadan. It was the pride of the Order at the time.

Richard Finn, an old friend from my first trip to Nigeria in 1960, was the local bishop. He had opened St Marys in 1964, and there is no doubt that another hospital was badly needed in a city that was bursting at the seams with an unprecedented explosion in its population.

Richard retired later to a little bungalow in Knock where Doreen and I were frequent visitors. He always had tea and cakes ready for us and inevitably the conversation would turn to Nigeria before we got up to go. There is an invisible bond between all those who have served on the missions in any capacity which binds them together in a way that is special, warm and deeply sentimental.

For there was always a welcome in a Mission Station. There was such a vast network of mission hospitals and schools that one automatically stayed in the 'mission house' when travelling. Sometimes we would stay in Protestant Mission houses if there was no Catholic Mission in the neighbourhood or if the Catholic one was full. This was a happy interdenominational practice that was reciprocated fully by both sides. Of course, there was no question of any charge.

In this way, practical ecumenism was far ahead of anything in Europe or America and you could travel the length and breadth of Africa going from one mission house to another for the cost of a small voluntary donation at each stop. Sometimes travellers – especially backpackers – abused this privilege, but in general it was respected and fully appreciated.

Four of us travelled from Mile 4 to Ibadan. We were a motley crew.

First, there was Sean MacCormack, a Kiltegan priest, who served in the Ogoja diocese for 33 years and who was known universally by the unflattering nickname 'MacMuc'.

MacMuc was a big florid Irishman typical of the colonial breed. By that I mean he was a hard man with a kind heart. In fairness there was no taint of racism in him, yet he was demanding on his houseboy and cook. Old coasters like MacMuc were of a special breed: tough, fair and determined. That was how they survived and how they got things done I suppose.

The second was Carla Simmons, the MMM in charge of the community at Mile 4. She encased herself in a practicality that helped protect her from the many jibes and insults that she encountered, not only because she was American, but also because she was an American sister in an 'Irish' Order of nuns. Carla was good company and I was to get to know her better when our paths crossed in later life. And then there was Mary, my daughter, a young Dental Student, and myself.

We loaded up our transport, a closed four-wheel drive pick-up, the night before.

The Sisters made sure we had sufficient bread, eggs, thermos flasks, tea, sugar, powdered milk, sandwiches and an assortment of fruit, mainly bananas. MacMuc checked the tyres, the brake fluid and the engine oil and filled our tank with diesel. Mary and I each packed a case for home and secured them with stout twine.

There was a goodbye meal for Mary and in the Convent in which the highlight was an iced cake with two lighted candles. Unfortunately, the candles somehow slipped and the melted wax made some of the icing uneatable. But everyone laughed and pronounced the cake delicious. We went to bed early but slept badly since we were due to leave before dawn. MacMuc had told us that we must start early for we needed to have some daylight left by the time we got to Ibadan, a distance of almost 700 kilometres. You may have guessed it. MacMuc was the last of the four to get up that morning.

By a two to one vote (Mary abstained) I was elected driver. This was not what I wanted as I had driven hardly at all in Nigeria since 1960. I had no license and no insurance and did not know the way. Furthermore I knew we would meet road-blocks when crossing the Niger River. And of course the driver is the one they pull out for questioning and from whom they demand *dash* (a small bribe). To make things worse, it was the rainy season so that we could expect flooded roads and swollen rivers. However, there was nothing I could do about it and I duly took the wheel.

Our trip went smoothly as far as Onitsha, the great market town on the Niger. Here we met the first roadblock. One is always apprehensive when coming to a roadblock. The soldiers lounge about all day, bored by the long idle hours, and only stimulated when they can extract money or goods from the occasional car or truck that comes along. Generally they wave white people on without too much hassle but sometimes they can be very aggressive and demand all kinds of papers. This is more so towards evening when they are often a little drunk, but we were approaching in daylight and were hopeful that they had not started on the palm wine yet. Nonetheless we were not sure what would happen.

A soldier thrust his Uzi or Kalashnikov (unlike modern day writers I do not know the difference) through the passenger window, and his colleague on my side demanded papers. I reckon our collective hearts beat a little faster. They stared hard at the four of us, but Carla had put on her nun's veil, and MacMuc his priest's habit, and this evidence of their calling seemed to convince them that we were ok. In any event I am not sure the soldier on my side could read the papers I handed him, unless he could read upside down!

Amid grins and much well-wishing – with MacMuc babbling away in the local dialect and giving each of them a blessing – we went on our way heading towards Benin City.

First we had to cross the Niger River, that great West African River in which the 35-year-old Scottish explorer Mungo Park drowned in 1806. But we weren't thinking of Mungo Park at that moment. We were merely intent on crossing the bridge and getting on our way before more soldiers stopped us.

As it happened our crossing was unremarkable, the bridge was intact, no one followed us, and we breathed a collective sigh of relief as we set our sights firmly on getting to Benin City.

It was in Benin City that Mary a month earlier had visited a local goddess. The goddess was a real live person who lived in a kind of shrine to which people could come, pay their respects, and have their futures told. She would, if they asked, cast a spell on an enemy or promise a good harvest. All or any of these boons she dished out depending, I suppose, on her mood and on the amount of money you paid her.

This time we went through Benin City without a stop and headed off on a brand new road to Ibadan. This road was beautifully tarmacked, straight as a die and was, *mirable dictu*, without a single pothole. Alas our dreams of getting to Ibadan early were suddenly dashed. For there, looming in front of us, like the Berlin Wall, was a pile of rubble, ten feet high. I pulled up sharply, and climbed up what was obviously a man-made obstacle. It came as no surprise, but nonetheless it was a shock, to realise that the road ended here. Ended in the middle of nowhere, and was impassible.

Around we turned and sped back towards Benin City, looking for the first exit that might take us to Ibadan. Sure enough we had barely travelled a couple of miles when a tattered sign nailed to a tattered pole pointed the way to Ibadan. We veered on to a *murram* (laterite) side road, on which we bumped our way forward, lurching from side to side. MacMuc was knocked off several times from a makeshift bed, on which he was attempting to sleep, in the back of the van. He was not amused. For my part I kept on driving and ziz-zagging in an effort to avoid the worst of the potholes.

It was now insufferably hot, and rain started to fall, which added to our misery. We did not stop to eat but munched away at our sandwiches not caring much what was in them.

We had travelled perhaps twenty miles on this awful road when we met our next problem. The rains had swollen a small river into a fast flowing torrent and we were confronted with crossing it without the aid of a bridge. There were several trucks and cars and lots of people standing talking in small groups on both sides of what was now a deep, fast flowing river, squeezed into a kind of mini gorge. I stopped and got out to see the lie of the land.

What I saw was not very reassuring. The locals had cut down two large trees and let them fall across to the other side. They had then placed planks cross ways and lashed them to the tree trunks. This was the bridge I was supposed to cross. The span of the 'river' was only about 30 feet, but what really scared me was seeing a truck sitting squarely in the waters below. Others had clearly tried crossing here and had come to a sticky end. It was still raining heavily.

I am not a particularly brave person, not often foolhardy, but this time I felt I could make it. My passengers seemed unable to say yes or no. However, before attempting to cross, I asked everyone to get out and walk across. They got out reluctantly and made their way to the other side safely, and then stood there waving at me to get moving. They were drenched at this stage and I am sure they were impatient to get out of the rain.

So, without much thinking, I drove slowly to the water's edge. Here a crowd of locals had gathered and started to clap and shout as I slowly moved across the wooden planks. I reached half way, the point of no return, when the planks started to rattle ominously. I was tempted to close my eyes but I knew that would be disastrous. Another group of locals, on the other side, waved me on with much gesticulating and all kinds of contradictory advice which I ignored. I went forward inch by inch, absolutely conscious that any slip on my part, any little misturn of the steering wheel or any wobble of the 'bridge' would see me tip over into 8 feet of water. I was perspiring from fear as well as from the oppressive heat by the time I reached safety on the other side.

Once over, I stopped while the others scrambled in, and then I revved up the engine and sped off as fast as I could, all the time waving to the people, on both sides of the gorge, who had guided us to safety.

It was about 6 p.m. when we reached the outskirts of Ibadan. Here we were met by another road block but this time I presented myself as a 'Reverend fadder' and we were duly waved on without any searching or any demand for a dash. Reverend fadders had a special place in the estimation of Nigerians that you may find hard to explain. I think the Nigerian knew that the Reverend fadders and Reverend sisters were not out to exploit them; that they were 'lifers' who actually loved Nigeria, and that they had dedicated their lives to helping Nigerians in hospitals, in schools and in the villages.

Ibadan itself consisted of a multitude of corrugated tin roofed shanty houses and, apart from the main thoroughfares, its roads were unpaved. They all seemed to be lined with deep open drains that stank to high heaven. It appeared to me quite unchanged, only larger than when I lived there twenty years earlier. *Plus ça change, plus c'est la même chose.*

I do not know what it is like today, but in those times, it was said to be the largest black city in the world. Yet it felt like home to me.

As I entered the city memories of 1960 crowded my mind. I thought of the hospital where I had worked and the long wards where I had spent many hours. The ghosts of so many of my African colleagues who had died in the Biafran War seemed to come out of the shadows and greet me back as an old friend. I thought especially of Ralph Eruchalu, Charlie Wokoma and Felix Udeh. I wondered if they were watching me. I hoped they were.

But to my story. We reached the suburb of Eleta at dusk. Darkness was descending swiftly now like a curtain coming down on a stage set. Myriad lights from candles, tilly lamps and open fires flickered and spluttered and threw a ruby hue over the fading city. We were tired and thirsty, hungry and happy all at once. But most of all we were glad to get out of the pick-up and stretch our cramped limbs. We had lived through a tough day.

Finally, as we rolled into the forecourt of the St Marys hospital, it stopped raining.

We had arrived.

CHAPTER 8

1979:
CAMBODIA/'KAMPUCHEA'

A Tragedy Brews

The origins of this tragedy are rooted in the defeat and with-
drawal of France from French Indochina in 1954. However,
independence brought no relief for the majority of Cambodians who continued to live in poverty and in subservience to
the ruling classes.

Consequently, a new breed of Cambodians emerged
anxious to change things for the better, and among these
was a young peasant called Pol Pot. He was a clever boy and
easily won a scholarship to study in Paris, but while there,
he embraced radical Marxism to such an extent that he was
expelled from France.

On return to Cambodia, he joined the outlawed Communist Party and fled to the jungle. Here he mobilised a band of
fanatical young people, the Khymer Rouge, who, aided by the
North Vietnamese, started a guerilla war to establish a New
Order. The regular army, controlled by Cambodia's leader,
Prince Sihanouk, fought back and was aided by US-led forces.
The conflict escalated. Soon B-52 bombers rained death and
destruction on the land beneath. Meantime the fighting grew
more intense and thousands of people were killed by both
sides. The world watched on impassively.

By 1970, the United States got fed up with the efforts of Prince Sihanouk to halt Communism and replaced him with Marshal Lon Nol in a bloodless *coup*. This angered the Prince who duly switched allegiance to Pol Pot and the whole shambles ended with the triumph of Pol Pot and the Khymer Rouge.

America walked out of Cambodia in 1973 and finally quitted Indochina with the humiliating fall of Saigon in 1975. It had taken them all this time to realise the futility and the cost in human suffering of their intervention. Ultimately the financial cost, and the growing impatience of the American people with armed intervention, forced the US authorities to do a U-turn and leave.

In the succeeding chaos, Pol Pot could now embark freely on his human experiment of creating a Marxian-based agrarian utopia in Cambodia. Cities and towns were emptied and everyone was put to work in camps in the countryside. Special purges were carried out against the educated classes, against Buddhist monks, Muslims, Christians, Chinese and against all minorities. Working hours were set from 4 a.m. to 9 p.m. Beatings, killings, torture and starvation were the rule. Millions died, millions fled and millions went missing. Even the name of the country was changed to Kampuchea.

The incredible excesses of Pol Pot and his fanatical Khymer Rouge regime could no longer be hidden in which, as usual, the innocent suffered the most.

In a strange twist of fate it was the North Vietnamese, now in a united Vietnam, who got rid of Pol Pot. They were hardened fighters and easily overran a chaotic Kampuchea where most people supported the invasion. And so, in 1978, a puppet regime of Kymer Rouge defectors was installed in Phnom Penh.

In a superb irony Pol Pot fled and gained sanctuary in Thailand, a country he had belittled and sneered at all his life.

He died twenty years later before he could be brought to trial in The Hague.

Although stories of Pol Pot's atrocities had been spotlighted on TV, it took Sydney Schanberg's reports in the *New York Times* in 1975 to make Western governments sit up and realise what was happening. Yet most ordinary people only became aware of these events after Christopher Hudson published *The Killing Fields* in 1984 in which he described Schanberg's escape from Kampuchea. After the award winning adaption of the book into film, virtually everyone in the civilised world became aware of Pol Pot and of what he had done.

I Go with Concorn

The small organisation called 'Africa Concern', which I had known during the Biafran War, has by now developed into a worldwide humanitarian aid organisation known as 'Concern International' or simply as 'Concern'. The founders, John and Kay O'Loughlin-Kennedy and Fr Raymond Kennedy, John's brother, appeared on the same platform urging the Irish people to support a new venture, aid to the victims of Pol Pot. As usual the Irish people responded generously.

The Finucane brothers, Aengus and Jack – both Holy Ghost Fathers – had always vigorously supported Concern and it was largely due to my admiration for them that I volunteered to work in Kampuchea in 1979.

By this time, TV was keeping us abreast of everything that was happening in the world, be it a volcano, a typhoon, a forest fire or a famine. The TV footage we saw of Pol Pols victims would move the hardest heart. So it was more difficult for me to stay at home than to go and actually *do something* that might directly help people.

The team that went included another medic, Dr Joe Barnes. I had known Joe Barnes since my intern days in the Mater hospital in Dublin when he had been one of my Consultants. I had always liked him and was delighted that we would be together.

And so the two of us travelled there in late autumn 1979 hoping to help in whatever way we could.

It was my first experience of the 'Far East' and I was filled with excitement as our plane landed in Bangkok airport. Asia is completely different to Africa and I was not prepared for the masses of people, the different dress and the ferocious traffic that I encountered on the way into the city.

Michael Fingleton, from Irish Nationwide Insurance, was sitting beside me on the plane. He was on the Board of Concern and a handsome donor, and he was coming to see what exactly Concern was doing. We spoke freely to each other on the plane, and I found him an amiable and interesting companion who was moved greatly by the sufferings of the ordinary people of Kampuchea. I was sorry to see how things went for his financial empire during the recession but I am no judge of these matters.

John O'Shea, a sports journalist with the Irish Press, had started his charity GOAL in 1977 and was also on the plane. I got to know John later when I worked with GOAL in South Sudan.

A Concern representative met the plane on the tarmac and took Michael Fingleton, Joe Barnes and myself directly to our hotel. He had a car waiting outside and we followed him gratefully without even getting our passports stamped.

The car was a smart Japanese one with air conditioning and a grinning driver who spoke no English but who was clearly delighted to have such important passengers. Once started, he switched up the volume of the radio so that any talk was impossible which suited us fine for we were absorbed in the panorama that opened before us as we negotiated our way through a maze of streets and alleyways. All were thronged with people, bicycles, carts, cars, buses and 'tuk-tuks' (motorised rickshaws) but we finally entered a quiet street and pulled up at a drab building simply named the 'RS Hotel'. The grinning driver carried our bags into the lobby and then disappeared who knows where.

Later we found out that most of the hotel patrons were humanitarian or UN workers like us but there was a fair sprinkling of sex tourists as well.

This was the first time I had seen overt debauchery. It took place in broad daylight even in the lounge of the hotel. Middle-aged European men were cavorting with beautiful Thai girls in plain sight, not waiting to do what they wanted to do in the privacy of their rooms. It was obvious too that some of the Thais were young men catering to the tastes of homosexuals.

The whole idea of this going on in the midst of the suffering we were expecting, appalled, disgusted and shocked me.

However, we were tired after the long journey and all of us were anxious to get on the road, so our thoughts were focused elsewhere and, for sure, on better things.

In fact, we were only two nights in the RS before being given some *bahts* (local money) and told to get on a local bus which would take us to the Concern camp at the little town of Aranyaprathet, near the Kampuchean border.

Michael Fingleton stayed on in Bangkok but Joe Barnes and myself set off, wondering what lay ahead.

Bangkok to Aranyaprathet

The bus trip was long, hot and boring. No one spoke during all the long hours we travelled and everyone seemed completely absorbed in his or her own thoughts. I was lucky in that I had a window seat, but there was little to see except peasants working in paddy fields.

I had brought a large bottle of water as I was told that it would be hot and that no stops were allowed. Hence my misery when I had a 'call of nature' which kept getting more acute as the miles rolled by. The more I tried to dismiss the urge, the greater it became. I was soon desperate. The empty water bottle provided my only chance of relief. I waited until those near me were either sleeping or had their eyes closed, and then, using my brief case as a cover, I surreptitiously relieved myself – as soundlessly as possible.

I will never know if anyone noticed. Perhaps, they wondered where I got the bottle of lemonade I was clutching when I finally stepped out of the bus!

We arrived at our destination in the late afternoon and were met by a young Thai man wearing a Concern T-shirt. He was a small stocky fellow who had a constant smile on his face and a ready answer to every problem. He led us to a white painted UN pick-up and drove us, perhaps half a mile, to the camp.

It was my second experience of refugee camps and I could see that they had improved little since my time in Biafra. There was the usual duplication of services by willing but inefficient non-governmental organisations (NGOs), the usual waste of money on projects – purportedly to help refugees – but which were both unsustainable and completely inefficient – and the usual rivalry between NGOs, many of which seemed more interested in gaining media attention and in fund raising for themselves than in actually helping people in distress.

For in distress these poor souls were, the harrowing stories they brought back from the 'killing fields' beggared belief. Most, probably all, had psychological scars but our concern was primarily with malnutrition and physical disease. We were not then aware that the psychological damage was as great as the physical damage. That realisation only came many years later in other wars and in other natural catastrophes.

Joe Barnes and I shared the same tent and so I got to know him very well. He had worked in Nigeria, in Osiomo, a leprosy settlement in Nigeria, some years before, and thus we shared stories of our lives in West Africa. One evening we fell into talk of our own families.

He told me that he originally hailed from Northern Ireland – in fact, he never lost his northern accent. He explained to me that he was a refugee. His family had been 'driven from Belfast' because they were Papists. Yet he bore no resentment against the Unionists and was in fact proud of his Belfast heritage. Now he lived and worked in Dublin but never forgot his real roots.

Like me he had always wanted to work in Africa and on returning to Ireland from Nigeria had been appointed a dermatologist in the Mater Hospital in Dublin. He loved his adopted home, but again, like me, he yearned secretly for the sun and colour of Africa and for the gaiety and warmth of the African people.

My recollection of Joe on the Thai-Cambodian border in 1979 was of a person completely at peace with himself and who delighted in doing all he could for the refugees in a quiet gentle way.

I used to say to him, 'I despair Joe; we are not really doing much good here. We are only seeing those ready to die or else just weighing babies and doling out multivitamin tablets.' Joe would smile at my frustrated eagerness and say 'Dom, we are here, aren't we?' How do you answer a question like that?

I have met Joe and his late wife Betty on and off over the succeeding years and, like so many others, have grown to respect, admire and love him. Doreen and I last met him in the Mansion House at a Refugee Trust (now Vita) celebration in 2014. He was then over 90 years of age and very deaf, but we talked quite a bit together, and he sent me a very lovely letter afterwards saying how much he enjoyed meeting up with Doreen and me again and encouraged me to keep supporting the 'forgotten poor'. Joe died shortly afterwards.

I Return Home Prematurely

My own trip was curtailed because of the sudden death of my brother-in-law, Joseph Hoade. He was returning home to Moycullen, a small village near Galway, on a dark wet night, after giving a lecture to farmers in Castlebar, the major town in County Mayo. Between the rain, the dark, and the fatigue he veered slightly and crashed into a vehicle badly parked on the side of the road. Joseph, better known as Joe, was an agriculture instructor and was extraordinarily popular because of his easy going ways and his soft humour. He had taught in St Patrick's College, Calabar for many years, before returning to Ireland, and Doreen, his sister, my wife, was especially fond of him. His death hurt her beyond measure.

Some families get more than their fair share of grief. His widow Rita brought up four children unaided, but her eldest son Joseph junior died after being struck by a car in Salthill, Galway, and her only daughter, Maura, died of a heart attack in her early thirties. Sadness has softened not soured her, and it is a tribute to her character that she manages to bring consolation to those who need it rather than look for any sympathy for herself.

As I was leaving Bangkok to fly home for Joe's funeral Alex Tarbet, the CEO of Concern, gave me an envelope to open on the plane. It contained £500 and a note saying 'Thanks for coming to help us.' The money was in notes, fresh crisp fivers! Naturally, I was delighted with this unexpected gift. I certainly could use it.

It was typical of Alex to think of others' needs. I am sure that he could have spent this money on himself. Sad then when he was later indicted for embezzlement and humiliated publicly. I don't believe Alex ever used a penny of Concern money for his own purposes. He was just a nice guy who was a bad bookkeeper.

My visits to Southeast Asia since those days have consisted of a few days stop-over on the way to or from Australia. It is now a thriving and prosperous part of the world thronged with tourists from the West.

Yet the scars of Pol Pot and his mad regime will take a long time to erase from the peoples psyche. If ever.

CHAPTER 9

1983: UGANDA

Perhaps, it was the disappointment at having to abort my trip to Cambodia or more likely the fact that I received undeserved payment which made me revert to my original goal of offering my services free to a mission hospital where I could fill in for someone and give a holiday to a tired mission doctor. I picked St Francis Hospital in Kampala, the capital of Uganda. It is better known as Nsambya hospital because it is situated near the top of Nsambya Hill, one the many hills in that city.

I have gone to Uganda several times since. My first visit in 1983 was the start of a love affair with that country and its people.

The Country

The great explorer Henry Morton Stanley – not Winston Churchill – originally described Uganda as the 'Pearl of Africa'. And he was absolutely right. Uganda is a glorious treasure lying deep in the warm heart of Africa.

Geographically, it is completely landlocked. You can see on the map of Africa that, roughly speaking, South Sudan is to the north, Kenya lies to the east and Tanzania to the south. Then three countries – Burundi, Rwanda and the DCR – complete the circle on the west.

Lake Victoria, Victoria Nyanza in the local Bantu language (Nyanza lit. lake), is an inland sea that sits like a bull's eye in the middle. I suppose, it has retained the name John Speke gave it in 1858 because no one country dared name it after any of its own heroes for fear of antagonising the others.

But apart from Victoria Nyanza, there are many other large and beautiful lakes within a days drive of Kampala, such as Lake Edward, Lake Wamala and Lake Kyoga. It's as if these masses of water have been scattered around just to delight the weary traveller.

Sometimes you come across a breathtaking spectacle such as the Murchinson Falls or the rapids at Jinja. At other times, you are enthralled by dark forests, towering mountains, wild national parks and game reserves – enough to overwhelm the senses.

Yet, not content with all this, Nature has blanketed much of the land in lush tropical savanna and dotted it with flowering trees, graceful palms, tall tamarinds and impenetrable masses of bamboo. The most striking trees – for me – are the purple flowering *Jacaranda* and the scarlet *Flame of the Forest*, while everywhere one finds multicoloured *bougainvillea* and deep red *hibiscus*.

As if forests, lakes and flowers were not enough Uganda hosts a rich and exotic fauna. If you open your eyes you will see tropical birds and butterflies often flaunting iridescent hues that defy description. And if you want wildlife, then it is there in abundance. Indeed not long ago the countryside was alive with antelope, zebra, lion, leopard and giraffe.

Of course, wildlife was far more plentiful some years ago. This was explained to my daughter Danielle and me by some elderly missionaries whom we met in Mbarara in 1992. Mbarara itself is a town roughly half way between Kampala and Fort Portal on the Rwandan border and is an ideal stopping off point when journeying to western Uganda. We were passing through and stopped to pay our respects, a typical 'colonial' thing to do. The elderly fathers there told us that when they came to Mbarara first, it was common for leopards to creep into town at night in search of food – including humans. They told us too of the many nights they crouched in the shadows outside the mission waiting to shoot a man-eater. All this was within living memory.

Those days have gone, but the national parks are still home to the 'Big Five' of Africa; the lion, the leopard, the elephant, the rhino and the buffalo. In addition to these you find giraffes, antelopes, ostriches, zebras and hyenas, and snakes – many of which are deadly.

But it is the birds that strike you most of all. They are colourful and noisy and beautiful, even the common African starling is beautiful. They soar, they twitter, they sing, they warble. No wonder the crowned-crane is the emblem of Uganda.

Unfortunately, the tropical climate and rich water supply make a natural habitat for all kinds of flying arthropods, including mosquitoes and tsetse flies. Many of these carry malaria, dengue and sleeping sickness. Indeed, it is a little known fact that the Zika virus was first discovered in Uganda as long ago as 1947.

It is a shame to visit Uganda and meet its people without knowing something of what has shaped the country. Like most outsiders I knew little about Uganda when I first arrived except that it had been ruled by Idi Amin, a tyrant by all accounts.

Uganda 1983

In 1983, Uganda was in turmoil. War raged in many parts and Milton Obote had just launched Operation Bonanza, in which his troops used a scorched earth policy, particularly against the Acholi people of the north. Fighting only ended with the triumphant entry of Museveni's National Resistance

Army (NRA) into Kampala in 1986 – three years after my visit. Museveni actively opposed Obote throughout and eventually, after much bloodshed, became President and has ruled continuously from 1986.

The Sisters had warned me that bloodshed had been almost continuous since independence, and that I would be virtually confined to the hospital compound – for my own safety. However, I did not tell my wife Doreen that there was any danger. In fact, I believed that the Sisters were probably exaggerating things.

I was soon to find out for myself that the country was in ruins; lawlessness was rife, murders and robberies an everyday occurrence and the economy was in tatters.

The Sisters were right.

Arrival at Entebbe Airport

There is an unfailing thrill in descending into Entebbe as dawn breathes life into a new day. You have just crossed the Sahara with its endless undulations and trackless sandy wastes. The waters of Lake Victoria begin to sparkle in the rays of the rising sun and here and there you see little plumes of smoke indicating that people are already stirring and that life is resuming its inevitable course for another day.

Before our plane even came to a halt there was the usual rush to stand up, stretch over one's neighbour and open the overhead lockers. The smart ones remained sitting, as they knew it would take a while before the doors finally opened. Anyway First Class passengers would disembark first, and the rest of us would just have to wait our turn.

I knew I was to be met at the airport and that took much of the stress out of the procedure. I also knew that there was no point in rushing these things. No one was ever yet left behind on a plane or stranded forever in an arrivals hall. Nonetheless, anything may happen when you arrive, tired and friendless, into a country where civil unrest, poverty and corruption are rife.

Thoughts on Arrival at a Foreign Airport

The pale-faced haggard-looking and obviously lost foreigner makes easy prey for scammers and tricksters and criminals who haunt the arrival hall in many countries.

But, apart from them, there are the usual obstacles to be overcome which require a steady head and above all patience.

For example, you are always confronted with the ordeal of immigration. This can vary from an endurable discomfort to a nightmare. You will usually find that you have filled the wrong visa form or incorrectly filled out the proper form or there are no forms to be found. In some Middle Eastern countries, the forms are completely in Arabic and you are left wondering what to write and where to write it. Signage may be in the local language only and it is easy to join the wrong queue. Ultimately, this entails going back to the end of the correct queue and starting all over again. In the meantime, you see lots of people ignore the whole process and march right up to the head of the queue and sail gaily on.

Once you get through, minus whatever number of dollars they may decide to extract from you (not in Entebbe) you must find your luggage. Luggage may or may not arrive, and often, if it does arrive, it is either after a long delay or arrives with locks broken and bags badly battered.

Having gone through Immigration and collected your bags you must then make your way through Customs. This can be just a matter of walking straight through while the customs officers examine other people bags. I have done this many times using strategic moments when the officials are distracted by something else. Well and good if it works. If not, then claim ignorance and say you did not understand what you were meant to do.

At last, you arrive in the arrivals hall proper. Hordes of placards face you with all kinds of names inscribed on them. You hope vainly to find your name and if you don't it is advisable to move on fairly smartly. Otherwise, you will be accosted by swarms of quasi porters, dubious taxi drivers and knowledgeable con men all wanting to carry your bags, all saying they will give you the best price into town and all claiming to be your dear friend.

You are tired, hot, sweaty, and overtly irascible by now. It is a moment when you are trying to make sure you still have all your things: passports, entry visa, contact numbers, money, water bottles, small bags, big bags, bags on wheels, bags with no wheels, bags with broken handles, bags that just won't roll properly. And you want to answer a call of nature.

That probably takes priority but first you have to find a toilet and take all your stuff with you. Mostly the toilets are dirty, there is no toilet paper, no towels, the floor is wet and you have to stand very far from the urinals, because each time they are used, people stand further and further away to avoid standing in the last man's urine. Of course, this evaporates in the heat and a sickly sweet smell arises wafting waves of little black flies upwards. And if this is not bad enough your nose is also assailed by the stronger more repulsive smell of stuffed toilet bowls. I do not know how ladies manage at all.

This is probably an unfair description of what many travellers experience in airports today but was surely the experience of many in the past.

Exit Entebbe Airport

In fact, Entebbe airport was quiet, almost deserted, when I arrived there in 1983. There were few passengers arriving, and customs and immigration officials were welcoming and were courteous. I passed through the dark cavernous arrivals hall and exited into blinding sunshine.

Wow, it is hot. But the fresh air makes me stronger and better able to dismiss the small persistent mob of hangers-on outside who pester me. This is easy. The people readily accept my waves of dismissal and do not physically intrude into my space as in some countries.

Yet I am more than 30 kilometre from Kampala and am not sure what to do next. Suddenly, a man approaches. 'You for Nsambya?' Thank God. This is great. 'Please wait. I bring the car'.

I stand there surrounded by bags and wait patiently until a noisy old Toyota pick-up trundles along and stops across the road. Sure enough it is my man. Thank God again. He has not forgotten me. The man from Nsambya gives a warm smile 'My name is Joseph. Welcome to Uganda.'

Joseph is very willing and helpful. He opens the boot and packs my bags in quite expertly, getting the maximum value from the minimum of space.

I do not care. This is great. Normally, I would be doubtful of getting in to a battered old Toyota, but now I don't care. I feel secure. Joseph bangs down the lid of the boot a few times until it is almost closed. Then he secures it with a bit of rope! I hold on to my purse and valuables – nowadays a laptop or iPod – but in 1983, a camera and an alarm clock.

And we are on our way. Joseph pays money at the exit of the airport and off we go towards the city. Huge billboards, show-ing the smiling face of the current, probably temporary, Head of State welcome us. And in many countries you pass under what I can only describe as a series of triumphal arches, either commemorating the country's independence or proclaiming, less gloriously, the fact that some congress or other is currently being held in the capital city. There were no arches on the road from Entebbe.

The road is a single carriage-way but smooth surfaced. Traffic is very heavy and progress slow. There are palm trees and banana groves aplenty on either side and, as one gets nearer the city, the number of cars, jeeps, buses, lorries, bicycles, pedestrians, taxis and military vehicles increase dramatically. There is much running and dodging as people cross the road causing us to brake violently on many occasions. The remains of many a vehicle litter the roadside with disquieting frequency, past victims of this bedlam. Horns are hooting continually now and you start holding on to your seat as Joseph swerves in and out of the traffic cursing volubly at other drivers.

Hawkers with trays full of useless knick-knacks come to the window every time the car slows, but the most amazing spectacle of all is to see pedestrians with huge loads on their heads weaving their way between buses and cars. Many of these are women who also carry babies on their backs.

After being immersed in heat, sweat, blaring horns, near misses and a kaleidoscope of colours and a cacophony of sounds, you expect to arrive at your destination. If it is a hotel there will be someone to open your door, take your bags and usher you into the semi-dark cool interior.

But not in my case. In my case, we drove up the pot-holed puckered Nsambya Hill past a school complex on the right-hand side where children in neat blue uniforms were playing outside. There was a line of stalls on the left-hand side, which dipped sharply down to a valley below.

Some of the stalls were loaded with pineapples, mangoes, paw paw and bananas, others offered skewered meat, live chickens, loaves of bread and raw meat – covered with flies – while yet others displayed electrical goods, notably batteries, purloined faulty video cassettes and every variety of wrist watch. Everything was on offer at 'very excellent prices'.

The hospital entrance is on the right-hand side beyond the school as you approach the top of the hill, and there are always rickety yellow taxis lined up in the vicinity. The taxi men, I discovered later, varied from truly honest souls to downright scoundrels.

The main entrance itself was not – nor is it yet – prepossessing. It consists of a crescent shaped, low one-storied building where people are checked in, registered and sent to the appropriate department once their paper work is in order. Throngs invariably mill about the semi-lunar space in front so that patients have to push their way forcefully to the various windows where they receive their passes to attend different departments.

We drove to the left past the gable end of the building and, after being waved through by security guards armed with rifles, we arrived at the convent, a two-storied drab grey building that housed the Sisters. At least, the convent had an air of calmness and serenity which eased a rising sense of apprehension that is part and parcel of any new venture.

Home Can be Anywhere?

We pulled up outside the convent on a patch of worn yellow grass. I was hardly out of the car when a Sister came out of the front door and beamed at me in a motherly way.

She said 'I'm Barbara...and you must be Dr Dom! ... You are so welcome....'

Barbara was a middle-aged English lady. I appreciated later that she had all the best qualities we associate with genteel English ladies, and were she not a sister she would have made a wonderful wife and mother. She had an unruffled manner and a gentle smile that oozed inner serenity and absolute faith in her calling. I got to like her more and more over the succeeding months.

'How lovely to see you. Welcome to Uganda … Do you want a wash before you eat? … And then you must rest….' She beckoned me follow her while Joseph unloaded the car and padded after us silently.

I was led into a large room on the left. It was clearly where the nuns ate, for there was a big wooden table in the centre with places set for perhaps eight people. There was an old-fashioned dumbwaiter, which took up half of one wall, and across from it against the other wall was an equally old-fashioned dresser, laden with blue Willow-pattern china. The bottom half was taken up by drawers, which presumably contained cutlery, tablecloths and all the usual accoutrements of a well-stocked dining room. Salt, pepper, ketchup and various cans containing tea and coffee and sugar were on a smaller table beside the dresser.

The whole atmosphere was cool and serene and inviting.

But what drew my immediate attention was the sumptuous spread, which was laid out on the big table. There were all kinds of fruits, a large bowl of salads, an inviting iced cake and lots of bread. The main meal was some kind of stew that was very good. Dessert consisted of ice cream and trifle.

I gathered that I would be eating lunch and dinner in the Convent but would be sleeping in the hospital. In fact, my sleeping quarters turned out to be a cordoned off area at the end of an outside corridor that ran the length of the main building. My 'room' was separated from the rest of the corridor by a temporary movable plywood partition which never closed fully. My inside wall was solid brick in which a window had been blocked off, my outside wall consisted of open trellised brickwork, which allowed lots of air to circulate but allowed lots of mosquitoes to come in as well. It also prevented any hope of privacy that I might have had.

But it was all they had for their visitor and I was happy to have a place of my own. I had arrived. I was home.

Nsambya Hospital, the Beginnings

When the Mill Hill Fathers came to Uganda in 1895, they concentrated their energies on setting up local Christian communities and on taking an uncompromising stand against slavery, which was still taking place unofficially. But they also saw the urgent need for Sisters to come and establish clinics and schools and lost little time in asking the local Franciscan nuns in Mill Hill to come and do so. The Sisters responded immediately, and so, on 3 December 1902, Sr Paul and five others left foggy London for the Dark Continent.

Young Sr Kevin, the future founder of the Franciscan Missionary Sisters for Africa, was among them. Little could this small group foresee the great hospital of Nsambya that would result from such a small inauspicious beginning.

Their arrival in Uganda on 15 January 1903 was like a circus coming to a small town. First, they were transported, from their steamship, the *Percy Anderson,* to the shore of Lake Victoria in 'gaily bedecked canoes' and then they were lifted 'shoulder high on brawny bronze arms and, amid the deafening clamour of drums, pipes and horns, sounding a vociferous welcome they were firmly dumped on the land that was to become their adopted country.' I quote from the 1981 'Souvenir Issue of Nsambya Hospital', which celebrated 75 years of service that year.

There is no doubt that the welcome was sincere. Even the Queen Mother of Buganda, the Namasole, personally welcomed the new arrivals as they made their way on the winding path to Kampala. The carnival atmosphere persisted all during the long trek. Eventually, they reached the mud and thatch convent prepared for them by the Mill Hill Fathers on Nsambya Hill. They arrived dirty, weary and exhausted.

Morning brought fresh hope. Within days, Sr Paul and Sr Kevin started a medical clinic under the shade of a mango tree. A mango tree that was to go into the folklore of future years. But they knew little of local diseases. Generously, the Cook brothers – committed Anglican missionaries – from Mengo Hospital, taught them tropical medicine and backed them up in every way they could. This gesture initiated a friendship between Catholics and Protestants that was to become a beacon to the rest of the Christian world.

Such was the inauspicious origin of today's Nsambya Hospital.

Nsambya Hospital 1983

The wards in Nsambya are long one-storied separate buildings, two for males, two for females, one for children, one for TB cases and one that houses maternity cases and the labour ward. They are all separated by well-worn grass patches and accessed from the outpatients, theatre and laboratories by concrete paths.

The nurse's block is separate and is a three-storied edifice situated to the back. It faces several small staff houses; there was always a group of hungry vultures between these and the nurses home, feasting on whatever offal and scraps of food that are discarded there.

None of the buildings could bear comparison to the multi-storied gleaming glass hospitals of the West. The wards were overcrowded, dark and dusty, the beds uncomfortable and the equipment was old and often faulty.

But Nsambya had a heart. Doctors and nurses *really cared* for their patients. They worked tirelessly and for little monetary reward. Patients supported one another in a way that is hard to explain, but was obvious to the outsider.

Although none of us on the staff were perfect, most tried as hard as we could, and amazing results were obtained with resources that were – even then – derisory.

There were also many simple non-medical differences between Nsambya and a Western hospital. For example, in the West, we bring fruit or biscuits or magazines to those we visit in hospital. But in Nsambya, if visitors brought anything, it was rice or a few mangoes or a bunch of bananas. In-patients were fed by their own families who squatted outside the wards for the duration of their stay. Relations set up temporary kitchens – and even temporary homes – on the grass patches between the different wards. Often they slept near their sick ones, lying on mats beside or under the beds. And this arrangement worked well. Patients were never lonely or isolated, they got the food they liked, and were part of the general gossip that buzzed around the hospital.

We also took it as normal, and thought nothing of the fact, that two or more patients shared the same bed or that some patients preferred to sleep under their beds while their relations slept on top.

In the paediatric ward, there was a kind of organised chaos with mothers and children everywhere, constant crying from babies needing attention and, overall, a thick sweetish odour of uncertain origin.

This would be dissipated every morning when all the cots were rolled outside and the ward scrubbed down with soap and water.

We had a small private wing in which wealthy patients paid for both their stay and treatment. It was to this unit that Idi Amin used to send some of his women to have their babies. Food was provided by the hospital for the private patients but, when I was there, I think the ordinary patients fared better.

I loved Nsambya.

Overseas Visitors

In peacetime overseas visitors, especially Canadian medical students and doctors, would come to Nsambya and bring gifts, money and modern expertise. It was a delightful, challenging and completely different experience for them and they would bring home numerous photos of medical conditions quite unknown in Canada.

Some of us viewed this as medical tourism. Perhaps we were jealous of the way many of our visitors lived. They generally lived in comfort, had the best of food and seemed to care more for doing procedures they would not be allowed attempt at home than for doing routine work. Yet this judgment is perhaps a bit too hard. They were certainly sincere and certainly generous, and these qualities were not lost on the locals.

Furthermore, these brief visits sometimes forged links with affluent hospitals overseas and occasionally an African doctor might get a placement in a top class hospital in America or Europe. Sadly, the majority of such placements resulted in the permanent loss of talented people from Uganda, which was quite the opposite of what had been originally intended.

Shortcut to the City

On quiet afternoons, I often made minor excursions into the city on foot. Mostly the reason was to visit a Forex to change dollars into Uganda shillings. I always used the shortcut, which entailed crossing the road at the hospital gates and passing between adjacent stalls and then unceremoniously scrambling and sliding down the side of Nsambya Hill. You crossed the railway line at the bottom and made the short climb up the other side of the valley. This left you right in the middle of the city and the whole excursion only took about fifteen minutes. Otherwise, on leaving the hospital you had to veer left and walk all the way down to a major roundabout, make a sharp turn right and head back towards town, a much longer journey.

When my colleagues heard that I used the shortcut they were quite upset.

Apparently, muggings, robberies, assaults and other nefarious activities were a daily occurrence along the valley path and no sensible person would use it. However, I was never molested. Indeed, I was helped by willing hands on more than one occasion when I slipped on a muddy patch or tripped over a hidden root.

Crossing the railway line was no problem. There were several rail tracks all of which were twisted and bent into grotesque shapes by bombs and mortar fire during the Tanzanian invasion and there were many sad looking railway carriages and derelict steam engines just sitting and rusting under the tropical rain.

Morning Rambles

My other minor excursions on foot were confined to very early morning, just before dawn, when I would go out the back gate, turn right past the parish church, and make my way for twenty minutes along a narrow track bordered by the homes of the local inhabitants.

Every house had its own little patch of ground in which a few skinny chickens or solemn-looking long-eared rabbits were kept. Paw paw, orange, lime, avocado and mango trees seemed to grow at random, although I am sure that each one belonged to a particular family. Banana groves were also interspersed between the houses with bunches of small green bananas clearly visible. They would ripen to a rich yellow and would taste far sweeter than any banana we get in Europe.

There were also many shrubs, bushes and trees – whose names I did not know – laden with exotic berries, which I am sure were good to eat.

During the day, there would be lots of children scampering about, mothers with babies at the breast and smaller infants on their backs. Women were seldom idle. They always seemed to be doing something, perhaps bent over a steaming cooking pot, or carrying a load of firewood, or going to or coming from the market. Always they were chatting to each other and almost always they were smiling.

At any time of the day a few dogs would always be slinking around searching for anything edible. Sometimes a golden jackal would come to town and join in the search for food. Dogs and jackals alike acted as useful scavengers ridding the place of rotting food waste as well as mice and rats.

Things were different in my pre-dawn walks. All was quiet except for the gentle rustle of leaves in a fitful breeze and the scurry of some animal prematurely disturbed from its slumbers by my approach. A soft night mist still blurred the outlines of anything further than 50 metres so that I seemed to be walking in a moving cocoon, where nature was at its kindest and where I was insulated from the real world with all its troubles and injustices.

Reluctantly, I would retrace my steps and face the reality of another working day.

Daybreak

I usually returned in time to join the Sisters for early morning Mass in the convent chapel. Sometimes, when I was earlier than usual, they were still at morning prayers, *lauds,* and I joined in, fumbling my way through psalms and canticles with which they were so familiar. The chapel was a long bleak whitewashed room with simple wooden pews on either side in which each sister had her own place. There was chipped statue of a weary looking St Francis at the back and a simple altar flanked by statues of Our Lady and St Joseph in the sanctuary. Fourteen painted pictures representing the Stations of the Cross hung on each sidewall, seven a side, third-rate paintings in which the images were all Italian looking. However, there was one concession to the local culture, the faces had been coloured black. I always think of Jesus as a dark skinned person but most cultures seem to have adopted him as having their own racial colouring and characteristics.

Sr Anne Scott, the American local superior, would always smile at me as I entered. I would slip in quietly and take a place at the back.

By the time Mass was over it would be quite bright and the new day had already begun in earnest.

Sometimes, if I were a little late, I would go to first mass in the parish church on my way back from my morning ramble. Here it was just like home with the same faces and the same few people occupying the same pews each morning. Initially we nodded to one another and later we smiled and bade the time of day, but eventually I would stop for a chat as we left the church.

Mass in the hospital chapel was also something special. This took place at 5.30 p.m. each day and was well attended by the hospital staff. The hospital chapel was just beside the main operating theatre and I think many of us slept through mass there after a long hectic day in the theatre next door.

Fr Semmanda was the hospital chaplain. We all loved him. He was an old man, 50 years a priest, and very holy. I think there is nothing more beautiful that to talk to a truly holy person. To be holy does not mean saying prayers all the time or following rigidly every rule of a religion. I think it means being humble, genuinely humble, caring for others and caring for them in a generous non self-seeking way. It also means being brave and speaking the truth and protecting the weak. Fr Semmanda had all of these qualities.

And in addition he was always smiling and always serene.

Mass in Africa

I have always had a special love for Mass in Africa. The congregation is much more involved than that in Europe or America. Everyone sings spontaneously and without the sort of self-consciousness that you find in Western churches, especially in Ireland. Even at an early weekday Mass, you will find a group of Africans beating native drums in a carefree happy way and all the time building up an atmosphere of expectation before the priest finally makes his entrance.

In Nsambya, people clapped hands at the elevation of the host and chalice during the holiest part of Mass. In Mozambique, I was surprised to find that everyone sat down during the reading of the gospel – an eminently sensible thing to do in my view. The sign of peace was always an important moment, during which people shook hands, embraced, or simply waved and smiled. I know this is difficult for many people for all kinds of reasons not least, in hospitals, for fear of spreading infection. But a nod or a smile or a little bow never harmed anyone.

In many parts of Africa, it is the custom that instead of passing a basket around, and so embarrassing some people, you drop your offering, usually a small coin, into a central basket while on your way up to receive holy communion. Of course, many simply march up at any time during the mass and give an offering.

The deep spirituality of Africans is very apparent in all aspects of African life and is a palpable reality when Africans join together to celebrate their Creator. Sunday Mass is a big weekly event for all the families. People gather well before starting time. Women are dressed in their best with gaily-coloured multi-patterned skirts, dresses and local costumes. They have flamboyant headwear, and their hair is set in all kinds of intricate plaits. Children are everywhere and add more noise, colour and confusion to the gathering crowds. The men wear spotless white shirts and long pants or dark suits. They seem to like shiny suits. Boys wear shorts and a T-shirt and girls wear party dresses.

Sunday Mass goes on for anything up to and beyond 2 hours. People come and go during the mass and no one is particularly bothered by the constant flux of worshippers. A stranger like me stands out like a sore thumb. Kids stare at me or smile shyly, especially, if I make a funny face at them. The very small ones scuttle behind their mothers' skirts.

The priest and or catechist drone on and on at homily time and I am not sure how many people are really listening. Homilies in Africa can be lengthy but then we all have plenty of time.

It is often unbearably hot and humid at Sunday Mass and either the fans do not work or you are so near a fan that it blows intermittent wafts of cold air right into your face which is most uncomfortable. That is when the electricity is working. Usually you are just left to sweat and endure hard wooden pews where the bit you kneel on is invariably too narrow or is so uneven that you must keep shifting your knees constantly.

After mass is over it is nice to emerge into the warm morning sunshine and face a bright new day. Lying in wait are the destitute, dressed in rags, and those disabled by disease such as polio or leprosy all hoping for some little help. I shamelessly had a pocket full of small coins to dispense on such occasions

I have been to mass in all sorts of places from the freezing north of the Arctic Circle, where the Northern Lights dance and glitter in the cold arctic sky, to Sydney where the Southern Cross rises each evening like a heavenly sentinel watching over our world. I have walked in the desert sun for many hours to get mass in the Belgian Embassy in Kuwait and have gone stealthily to mass in a back street chapel in Benghazi. I have been at mass on ocean liners, in the great basilicas of Rome, Lourdes and Paris but the Mass in Africa has a colour, sound and comradeship that is the most special of all.

Medicine in Nsambya

Immediately after Mass, I drink coffee and eat some bread before starting my day's work. Work can involve being in theatre all day or doing clinics where one may expect to see over 100 people or going around the wards and – in normal times – doing outreach or 'bush' clinics.

I soon get expert at doing Caesarean Sections with a personal record of having done eight in one day. For any expertise in this regard, I thank a Ugandan colleague, Joseph Adrigwe. Joseph was one of the gentlest, kindest and most skilful surgeons I ever met. He was a tall person, slim with long fine fingers. His voice was quiet and his manner courteous without being deferential. We became very close and shared many a theatre session, many a chat at night, and many an exchange of our hopes and fears.

I have tried in vain to locate Joseph since those days. Some say he died of natural causes, some say he was murdered because he was born in the north of the country – ergo an enemy of the southern Baganda – and some say he is somewhere in remote parts of central Africa.

Then there was Pius Okong, another tall African, but this time from a different tribe. Pius was a gifted obstetrician and was the kind of person always in good humour, always talking and always laughing no matter how tough things were. He later went on to the highest position in the Department of Health and has lectured both in Africa and in Canada. When my daughter Sallyann was a medical student in Galway, she spent a summer elective in Nsambya and worked under Pius. I think that this was a time when she did more sightseeing than medical work.

When Pius married, he called his first daughter Doreen, after my wife, and this is a signal honour, which quite often Africans give you as a mark of friendship.

Since I was so close to my African colleagues, both in the work place and at recreation, they naturally dropped their guard when in my company and I learned – despite instinctively knowing – that they could size up expatriates with uncanny accuracy. We had many a laugh together in the evenings and our shared lives bonded us together as a team that, for me at least, would always be unbreakable.

My two expatriate colleagues were both sister doctors.

One was Sr Miriam Duggan who hailed from Limerick. Miriam was a bundle of energy for whom nothing was impossible and nothing too great to tackle. She always spoke her mind and had no time for double talk or hypocrisy or backbiting. Physically, she was a small person with small nimble fingers and a sure way of doing things. If she had a fault, it was in expecting everyone to work as hard as herself and she had little patience with incompetence and none with laziness. Miriam never spared herself and set standards for herself that few could match.

She sometimes spoke of Bishop Casey of Galway who was from the same area, but her more important clerical connection was Pope John Paul II. She was within a few yards of him in May 1981 when Mehmet Ali Ağca shot him. She would smilingly confess that even she was stunned into inaction by that event.

Miriam eventually specialised in HIV-AIDS and was recognised by the Ugandan Government for her efforts to prevent and treat this scourge, which, unbeknown to us, was starting in 1983, during my time in Nsambya.

Sr Veronica Cotter was my other expatriate colleague. Veronica was from Cork and had been a brilliant student obtaining first place in her final medical exams. But more important than her academic achievements was the fact that she was a born diagnostician. The African doctors recognised her excellence as a doctor and we were often amazed at the way she could make a diagnosis in cases that had stumped us. Do you remember the TV series about the brilliant 'Dr House'? Well, Veronica would tie him in knots.

But Veronica had other qualities too that made her special. She was the kind of person you just want to tell your troubles to *and she would listen*, calmly pondering every word you uttered, and totally understanding everything you said.

Originally trained as a physician, she had become – like Miriam – an obstetrician and surgeon and paediatrician – all rolled into one. And, like the rest of us, she shared the on-call, one-in-three roster.

In addition to all that, Veronica took care of the medical administrative work, ran the private clinic for rich Ugandans (often for the military who did not pay), and liaised with the civil authorities on many issues.

Medical Haps and Mishaps

In my typical day in Nsambya, I came to accept things as they were, not as they should be. Unfortunately, part of the price one pays for being overworked and always in a rush is the making of unforced errors. There are two instances that stand out in my mind.

The first involved a sixteen-year-old boy who had a lump in his left groin diagnosed by the houseman as a possible TB abscess. It was scheduled last on the operating list for drainage, a simple enough procedure you'd say. The patient was rolled into the theatre and I decided to do the drainage myself rather than send for the houseman who was somewhere on the wards.

I scrubbed up in the minimum of water (as usual) and put on rubber gloves (recycled, rewashed and re-powdered many times, as usual), pushed open the swing doors (badly needed oil, as usual) and entered the theatre proper.

The theatre was housed in a small single-storied building beside the hospital chapel. The concrete path running beside the theatre was bumpy in places and this meant that patients were sometimes unexpectedly jarred as we pushed them on trolleys to or from the wards. The operating room itself was fairly small with two windows through which we could see passersby and they could see us. There was often a gentle breeze – after all the hospital was on the top of Nsambya Hill – and this was welcomed very much by all who worked in such a cramped space.

Mr Pius sat at the head of the operating table. Mr Pius – everyone called him 'Mr' Pius – was a local man who had gone to primary school and then learned to give anaesthetics under the guidance of a fully trained anaesthetist. He had an ether vaporiser EMO machine similar to the one I had used in Nigeria and was expert at using it. Mr Pius could also intubate, a skill that requires much practise.

I suspect that you can teach anyone to do almost anything given enough practise. Which brings me in mind of the late Des Kneafsey, a superb chest surgeon, who worked in Galway in the same hospital as me. Des once told me that you could train anyone to do heart surgery if you showed him how to do it often enough. I believe him. So it was no surprise that Mr Pius was an expert in using his EMO machine and was far more competent with it than any doctor.

Mr Pius seldom laughed, but it was worth waiting for the occasional smile when his whole face would light up and his eyes sparkle with unfeigned delight. We used his services for long cases, especially on the abdomen and chest. We also had him there to give a shot of pentothal and maybe pass a tube when we wanted to do something quickly such as drain a deep abscess, set a fracture or change a burn dressing. Otherwise, and for the most part, we used either local anaesthesia or spinal anaesthesia. We all got so proficient in inserting spinal needles that I used to quote Joe Costello, an anaesthetist friend in Galway who said that 'he could throw a spinal needle from the door of the theatre and get it in the right place in the patients back '

So in the case of my sixteen years old, I asked Mr Pius to give him a quick whiff and I'd lance the abscess. I painted the area in providine, and then draped a few green towels on the thigh just leaving the dome of the abscess swelling exposed.

There were two nurses also present, one we call the scrub nurse who would scrub up and assist at whatever operation you were doing, and another called the runner nurse, who was the 'go-for', who would do a swab count and fetch any extra instruments as required.

In this case, I did not need a scrub nurse so there were two runners in the room. I nodded to Mr Pius and he did his magic.

There are three things that always fill me with awe. First is seeing a baby emerge from the birth canal and start to cry, second is the sight of an aeroplane taking off into the sky, and third is the vision of a wide awake person suddenly becoming unconscious while you are injecting pentothal or propaphol. So I looked at the young man and then at Mr Pius who returned my nod indicating that I could now start.

I felt the lump briefly and noted it was warm. Not the typical 'cold' abscess one associates with TB. Must be a pyogenic one I reckoned. Then I noticed a definite sense of vibration – we call it a thrill – as I steadied the bump, with scalpel poised above it. I automatically presumed that the thrill was due to vibration transmitted from the underlying femoral artery.

And yet, incredibly, I did not cop on. I made sure my runner had a large kidney dish ready to collect the expected gush of pus, and then made my incision. I cut deep and boldly – and stupidly.

Horror struck me like a thunderbolt. There was no pus. Instead, a gush of bright red blood spurted up drenching my gown and splattering my glasses so that I could hardly see. Instinctively, I tried to stop the torrent by pressing down on the gaping incision.

My abscess had turned out to be an aneurysm, an abnormal dilatation of a blood vessel. In this case it was clearly an aneurysm of the femoral artery. I kept up the pressure with my hand while Mr Pius set up an IV line and we all waited impatiently for the second runner to bring us a bottle of blood from the makeshift hospital blood bank. I knew there were one or two bottles of blood there which we kept for obstetric emergencies. There was one bottle of O Rhesus positive blood but no Rhesus negative blood was available. I told Mr Pius to go ahead regardless. Our boy was now going into shock and I feared for his life. Once Mr Pius had got the blood transfusion going I felt a little easier. Just a little. Because more calamities were to follow.

Can you imagine how I felt when I straightened up from my bent position and struck my head against the glass blood bottle – blood was stored in bottles in 1983. But it was worse than that. I overturned the whole drip stand and the solitary bottle of blood that existed in the whole of Kampala came crashing down on the floor and smashed into a thousand pieces. I kept pressure on his groin for another ten minutes but every time I eased the pressure blood kept coming. I now feared the boy would exsanguinate.

I then did the only thing I knew that would stop the bleeding. I put a ligature around the torn vessel above and below the tear. This stopped the bleeding and his blood pressure started to climb back towards normal.

But I had now stopped all blood flow to the leg and I knew that, unless a bypass circulation had developed in the previous few months, the boy would lose his entire leg. Deprived of blood, the leg would become necrotic and he would lose most of it from *dry gangrene*. If it became infected it would become moist and smelly and he would lose it from *wet gangrene*. If gas-forming organisms got into the dying tissues he might get *gas gangrene*. If worry could kill then I was a dead man.

My patient was returned to the ward with his left leg elevated, and as many painkillers as I could afford to give him. The foot was swathed in towels doused in the coldest water we could find. I checked the colour of his foot and felt for an ankle pulse twice a day for the next ten days.

The more I read about tying off the femoral artery the more dubious I became about the chances of saving his leg. I kept my fears to myself. None of my colleagues mentioned it and I am sure I was naïve if I thought the news of what happened had not spread like wildfire throughout the whole place.

Finally, after ten days, I was myself again. The foot stayed viable, the pain subsided; an ankle pulse returned, the wound healed and the boy got up and walked on both legs. He never knew nor did he ever ask what all the fuss was about. He must have thought I was a strange doctor who came to see him twice a day while I barely noticed those in the beds on either side of him.

I often tell my students that I will write a book solely devoted to the mistakes I have made in my life as a doctor. I tell them mistakes will happen, but they have been warned and hopefully they will not repeat the mistakes I have made. So I implore all young aspiring doctors, to please, please take the time, even if it is only a few minutes, *to examine patients carefully* before sticking a knife in them.

However, there is one good case I should share. This involves a 33-year-old lady who came to us with persistent vomiting for no apparent reason. The vomiting was projectile in nature, just as one finds in a baby with pyloric stenosis – a narrowing of the outlet of the stomach. This lady was a nun, had grown up in South America, and was losing weight at an alarming rate. She had no pain, no blood in her stool and there was nothing special about her vomit except that it was getting progressively worse to the extent that she could no longer keep down any solid food.

I was unable to diagnose the cause and I really did not know how to handle the case apart from intravenous feeding. It was natural then that I would ask Veronica to see this patient. She agreed immediately. We all turned to Veronica when we were puzzled

There was nothing unusual on physical examination. A full blood count and serum electrolytes were normal. The urine was clear. All we could see was a huge loss of weight. She weighed not much more than seven stone (44 kilogram).

Veronica pondered for only a few moments and then decided she would do a barium swallow. 'There must be an obstruction in the oesophagus' she mused, 'Maybe this lady has cancer of the lower end. Let's do the barium swallow now.'

So off we went to the X-Ray Department.

Only simple X-rays for broken bones or, at the most, a plain chest or straight abdominal film had been done there for many years. Yet we found a bottle of barium, sticky white stuff. We stirred it up and added some water so that it would look like and flow like Hellman's Mayonnaise.

Then we brought our patient in and made her swallow the barium while Veronica took X-rays at 5-10 second intervals.

Lo and behold the white radiopaque barium was held up at the bottom of the oesophagus like sludge in a narrow funnel. There was no doubt about this being the place of the obstruction. Was it a cancer? No, the barium bolus in cancer of the lower end of the oesophagus typically ends in a rat-tail appearance, not the smooth round shape that was on our X-ray.

Veronica turned to me and said 'I should have guessed. If I had listened to her story of being brought up in South America I would have thought of it earlier'

'Thought of what?'

'Chagas disease of course'

'Oh' I am perplexed. Somewhere in my subconscious mind I remember the name Chagas. He was a Spanish guy...wasn't he? I vaguely recall the name 'Carlos Chagas' or was it Carlos Gorgas? It is something to do with South America all right. Some sort of tropical disease.

Veronica smiled indulgently at me.

'Carried by the kissing bug, a triatomine....' There was a wink in her eye when she pronounced the word kissing.

My memory sharpened. The kissing bug...lands on your face and bites you painlessly often near your lips. It carries the American variety of trypanosomiasis, a family of parasites that causes sleeping sickness in Africa. I was to see lots of sleeping sickness a few wees later when on my weekend break in Baluba.. The dreaded tsetse fly, common around Baluba, carries it and can even bite through your socks and pants.

But in South America chronic trypanosomiasis causes achalasia not sleeping sickness. In achalasis there is paralysis of the lower end of the oesophagus and destruction of the little nerves that control the lower sphincter so that food cannot pass through. As a result, the rest of the oesophagus between the pharynx and stomach swells up with fluid and food and the patient relieves himself – or in our case relieves herself – by repeated painless bouts of vomiting in which the vomited contents spurt out like a fountain. Projectile vomiting.

So we had the diagnosis. There is no medical drug or treatment that will cure Chagas disease. It needs surgery, in our case urgent surgery. But where could we send this patient? Mulago – the University Hospital – was in tatters, and flights out of Entebbe to South Africa, where very serious cases were sent in the past, were extraordinarily complicated and rare. We might have tried Nairobi. The Jomo Kenyatta Hospital in Nairobi is an excellent centre nowadays but was grossly overcrowded, understaffed and under-resourced in 1983.

Veronica hardly hesitated, 'We will do it together.'

I was non-plussed. This was major surgery. There was just Veronica and I to do the cutting and Mr Pius with his EMO machine to keep the patient asleep for perhaps two to three hours. We had no monitoring equipment, no apparatus to do blood gas analyses, no way to tell blood 'sats', little or no blood on hand for transfusion and only our own home made intravenous fluids of normal saline and dextrose saline.

'We will do it together. It has to be done.' She smiled at me, and yes, I felt perhaps we could do it together.

The big day came as inevitably all big days come. I should have been uptight and shaky but I was actually very calm. I had complete faith in Veronica and in the deft touches and skillful way she faced any difficult operation. Mr Pius was all business making sure his machine was working satisfactorily, filling syringes with Pentothal and muscle relaxants and setting up a lovely intravenous line in the patient's right arm.

We tilted the patient on her right side so that Veronica could get access to the lower oesophagus through the chest and that it could also be accessed from the underside of the diaphragm. I should have been thinking great thoughts, perhaps praying, but in truth I was too preoccupied with the task in hand to think at all.

The operation went smoothly. Mr Pius sat impassively at the head of the table only making eye contact with me when I looked directly at him. Yet there was always empathy between Mr Pius and myself. I still remember him with a sweet nostalgia after all these years.

Veronica's operation was a success and more importantly the patient made an excellent recovery. It was all in a day's work for Veronica but a momentous occasion for me. I kept one of her barium films to show students when I returned to Ireland.

I ask them 'What is this?' They mostly reply 'An obvious pyloric stenosis.'

I then tell them it is not a dilated stomach. They look incredulous.

'This is a dilated oesophagus' I almost smirk. 'A mega-oesophagus.' I pause for effect. There is silence. Because they know what is coming next.

'You are the pick of the Leaving Certificate classes in Ireland, so please tell me what is causing this?'

'I'll give you a clue. This is an X-ray of a 33-year-old woman from Brazil.'

They almost all say 'Achalasia'.

'And the cause of the Achalasia?'

'Idiopathic' they reply. Idiopathic means cause unknown. It is fashionable to say 'idiopathic' or 'autoimmune', or in cases of abdominal discomfort to call it 'diverticulitis' – like it was fashionable in Axel Munthe's *San Michele* to attribute all abdominal discomfort of unknown origin to 'colitis'.

Only one student in the RCSI has given me the correct answer in all these years.

After that dramatic encounter I feel you may be let down by the next case. But it is nonetheless instructive, and the patient was very thankful afterwards. It concerns an elderly man who came to hospital on a regular basis with abdominal pain, huge abdominal distension and progressive constipation. This was a case of volvulus, a twisting of a segment of large intestine, so that food and fluid and faeces and large volumes of gas accumulate with no means of escape. The pain of volvulus can be intense as the gut writhes and twists in a vain effort to uncoil itself.

Volvulus is more common in African countries than elsewhere, possibly due to a high fibre diet combined with an anatomical variation in the way the large intestine is tethered to the back wall of the abdominal cavity. Ideally we open the abdomen and uncoil the offending twisted loops of gut, and afterwards we fix things so that further twisting cannot occur. Sometimes we resect, that is, we have to cut out the offending loops, because of the danger of the gut perforating with subsequent peritonitis.

This man was far too old for a major procedure and so we merely tried to relieve his symptoms immediately – if only for a few months – by passing a long rubber tube up through his anus so that the trapped contents might escape and the gut uncoil harmlessly. There is always the danger that if one does not take great care the tube may rupture the colon with disastrous results. This was a hazard inherent in our treatment.

It happened that one day, around lunchtime, he presented once again with all his usual symptoms. I had finished my list and had asked the houseman, Dr Proszekia ('Pross' to her friends), to do a few minor cases and finish up by passing a rectal tube on our volvulus patient.

I was having lunch in the Convent and had hardly finished my soup when Pross came running in. I should explain that Pross was a tall, good-looking girl, very well connected in medical circles; her mother was the MO to the Entebbe airport and her uncle was a professor of Pathology in Makerere University, but most importantly – as far as I was concerned – she was a caring and conscientious houseman.

She was obviously upset. 'Dom, Dom' she cried 'I've lost the tube.'

'Hold on, hold on Pross… What do you mean you lost the tube? … Isn't there another one you can use?'

'No, no … I mean it is gone up. Out of sight … I … I can't see it….' Pross was really getting agitated. My aplomb was not helping either.

Then Veronica, sitting near me, started to laugh. 'For heaven sake Pross, stop worrying. It will be all right. This is not the first time that this has happened. Well, I mean that I have seen it in other patients, although not in this man. Come and have lunch with us. *Please*. Sit down and we will all go and see your patient with the lost tube afterwards.'

This calmed Pross. I needed calming too because I was not sure how I should or would handle this strange turn of events. Veronica laughed outright again. That calmed me.

And so we ate our lunch, perhaps more quickly than normal, but made no further reference to Pross' problem. We deliberately took coffee afterwards and listened to Sr Anne Needham (the hospital accountant) talking about the day she found a snake sliding across her office table. She said she had been terrified and sat there transfixed until the snake slithered down and out the door.

At this stage Pross was visibly getting uneasy, and clearly not interested in the snake story, so we all trooped down to the theatre. Our volvulus friend was lying fast asleep on the table, his belly was flat and the lost tube was lying harmlessly on the floor. He had expelled it and a considerable amount of wind and feces all at once.

We had a good laugh about this afterwards. Pross and I had learned something new that day, something we will never forget. I do not know what became of Pross afterwards.

Pross was brought up as a lady, shy and gentle and probably quite unsuited to the hurly burly of medicine in a hospital like Nsambya. But I suspect she made a great doctor.

The Start of AIDS in Uganda

It happened this way. Initially, there was only a trickle of patients, mostly adult males, which soon swelled to a flood, all presenting with severe diarrhoea and dehydration. There was no apparent reason for the diarrhoea.

Unlike cholera, the diarrhoea persisted and worsened despite rehydration and antibiotics. These men were almost all MSM – men having sex with men – but by no means could we categorise this as a male homosexual disease, because we soon began to see heterosexuals of both genders affected as well.

The sufferers usually came to our notice after trying a variety of ineffectual local remedies. When we saw them, they were weak and usually incontinent of feces. Sometimes they were carried in moribund.

Many too had coexisting conditions such as Kaposi sarcoma, thrush infections and refractory pneumonia which we thought were merely coincidences at the time.

Since almost all were grossly underweight a colleague, David Werrawada, in Makerere University, had named the symptom-complex 'Slim Disease' the previous year (1982). But we were no wiser as to the cause of the condition which was spreading like wildfire throughout Uganda and sub-Saharan Africa.

Someone noticed that most came from the Rakai district, on the shore of Lake Victoria, and so we assumed that there was some local factor, perhaps infected fish, that was capable of transmitting an unknown pathogen to humans. Several more years passed before the HIV virus was identified as the cause and even today it remains a dreaded condition despite the great recent advances in treatment.

Nine Years On: HIV Reigns

I jump momentarily forward in time to 1992. In that year, I was asked to do an AIDS survey for the WHO in Uganda. This time I took my daughter Danielle with me, and we made several trips with outreach AIDS teams. Danielle and I went into houses, nice houses from the outside, but which were rotten to the core inside with vomitus and feces everywhere. To crown it all, the head of the household would be lying on his bed, fully conscious but clearly dying and beyond our help.

Here we saw first hand the devastation that HIV-AIDS was causing to local communities. Whole villages were deserted and, since it was the 20–40 years age group that was most affected, it meant that old people were left to take care of their orphaned grandchildren, often up to 30 at a time.

The shocking practise of men seeking out innocent school-girls for sex was rampant. It was assumed that you could not get AIDS from an untouched virgin. But of course you could *give* AIDS to anyone. Many thought that mosquitoes were spreading the dreaded disease. Others blamed the transmission on infected needles. Yet others considered AIDS a curse from an outraged God. Even doctors were responsible for such misinformation. Fear stalked the land.

For us medics, the danger of getting the virus from patients was real, and one Dutch doctor not only contracted HIV but also actually died from it after doing a manual removal of a placenta in an HIV positive patient.

Miriam used to say that she could diagnose AIDS by a distinctive smell from a patient. I don't know about that, but I do know that there was a characteristic smell of decay, of rotting fungus and of stinking faecal matter from many of them, probably due to opportunistic infections or mere inability to cope with excretory body functions.

We tried to treat the complications of AIDS at our Wednesday clinics in the hospital. The United States Agency for International Development (USAID) provided much needed funds for medicines, clean linen, nourishing food and extra nurses to cope with the epidemic, and I make special mention of all those dedicated people, including the Scottish priest Fr Steve – *a père blanch*, who put their lives on the line, when they washed patients, cleaned houses and emptied the slops of the affected.

The Rakai

Neither Danielle nor I will ever forget our visit to the Rakai. It was a ghost place. Only old men and young children were left, and many of these sat listlessly around, just gazing across the blue, tranquil, but indifferent waters of Lake Victoria.

It was during this visit with my daughter that she was introduced to Nsambya's travelling Mother and Child clinics where we dished out folic acid, iron tablets and multivitamins to all and sundry. It was here also that the locals assigned Danielle and I to the care of the Antelope. Every family had an animal that watched over them. I am not sure how much protection we would get from an antelope. But this was the way the people thanked us and we were pleased. The nominated animal was supposed to have characteristics which his human protégés shared. Danielle and I could certainly run and that is surely a feature of the antelope. Clearly, they did not think we were brave like the lion or as swift as the leopard or as cunning as a snake.

I think it was in a village, *en route* to the Rakai, that Danielle and I first saw women making *matoke*. This is a traditional Ugandan food, which can be delicious or awful depending on how it is made and how long it is left to cook. In rural areas the large starchy banana (the cooking banana or plantain) is boiled and, while still hot, is wrapped in its leaves and buried in the ground where it is left to simmer.

This, for me, makes as tasty a *matoke* dish as you can get anywhere.

Breaks in Routine

During the three months of my 1983 visit, I rarely left the hospital compound for more than an hour or so.

My first official outing was to bring a comatose young man with a gunshot head wound on the short drive to Mulago Hospital. It was a journey in vain. Mulago was a shambles and the few brave doctors and nurses who worked there were exhausted and unpaid and fought a hopeless battle to save whatever lives they could, with hardly any drugs and with most of the equipment looted or damaged beyond repair.

My second excursion was to visit Butabika Mental Hospital, the major psychiatric hospital in Kampala. Again I was delivering a patient. The 'hospital' lay about twelve kilometre to the east of central Kampala, close to the shores of Lake Victoria, and I had no doubt that it was once a fine place. But all I saw was a bleak building from which the original paint had long since peeled, revealing streaks and patches of dun coloured brick beneath.

Today Butabika is the National Referral Hospital for mental health in Uganda and is a gleaming edifice worthy of any capital city.

Patients are treated using the most up to date methods and their accommodation is both clean and comfortable.

However, conditions in 1983 were quite different. In fact, appalling. Poorly clad inmates – I hesitate the call them patients – sat around outside, singly or in small groups, with vacant expressions on their faces. There was little talk between them apart for occasional incomprehensible mutterings. Those inside the building were even more pathetic. They were huddled in corridors and at corners, some with a dirty tee shirt and tattered shorts, others with no clothes at all. Some kept up a constant moaning while a few sat there, staring blankly, obviously living in some strange world of their own.

A few remained in dirty cells with absolutely no sanitary facilities. Some of them were still asleep on the stone floors when I went there. The air in the cells was heavy with human stench but I suppose these lost souls got used to it.

Everywhere I went, I was greeted by staring eyes, which followed my every move. Even the 'nurses' seemed lifeless. Indeed many could only be distinguished from their patients by their short white jackets.

There seemed to be no hope anywhere, and if despair was an object then surely you could touch, feel and smell it here.

When I revisited Butabika in 1992, I took the opportunity to stress the need to help the HIV-AIDS patients there. In this way, I hoped to get extra food and medical supplies for Butabika which would benefit all the patients, not just the AIDS ones. I wrote strongly:

'Patients here ...live on scraps, scavenge the 'warders' garbage and eat ants and crickets and any insects which they find in the grass or on their clothes.'

I believe that it moved the authorities to allocate more food to the hospital. Occasionally reports are actually read by someone who cares.

Miriam Duggan brought me on my third outing. It was typical of her to discommode herself for others and so she made time one morning to show me something of Kampala. It was raining heavily, but that did not deter Miriam who was hatless and coatless as she revved up the hospital pick-up and headed off to the town.

First, she brought me to the Kampala Mosque, since replaced by the huge Gaddafi Mosque on Kampala Hill. We climbed the minaret, or I should say I chased after her, up the winding stone stairs, to the top. Here we gazed at the city spread beneath us. She pointed out things that I could not see because of the rain and she gave me a breathless account of the doings of Idi Amin, Obote and Museveni – which I could not remember.

I pointed out politely that both of us were getting drenched standing exposed, but she dismissed my wimpy protestations by telling me 'What's a drop of rain...the sun will dry you off in five minutes.' She was right, of course. Miriam was the kind of person who would run where others walked.

We looked across the valley that runs through Kampala like a parting in a thick head of hair, dividing the city into two.

Romanticists have likened Kampala to Rome saying that both cities are built on seven hills. But, like Rome, this is a myth, as both cities have more than seven hills. Miriam pointed them out to me and named them, all of which I promptly forgot.

After this, she drove me to the Martyrs Shrine at Namu-gongo, fifteen kilometre from Kampala. Pope Paul V1 had visited it in 1969, the first papal visit to Africa. The shrine was just a circular wooden structure, like a large corral, with the centre, where the martyrs were burned alive, cordoned off by ropes.

It had a strange atmosphere as if the spirits of good and evil were unable to break away from the place of their confronta-tion. Nowadays, the site is covered with an impressive canopy from which I think the ghosts of the past will never escape.

My fourth outing was a weekend break in Baluba, on the northern shores of Lake Victoria. The same Joseph who had met me in Entebbe drove me in a borrowed Land Rover. But now I was an old hand and we talked easily and casually together. It was great just to get away from the confines of the hospital, the long low wards, the small cramped operat-ing theatre, the hectic labour ward and the endless stream of people who pushed their way into every out-patients clinic and who crammed the emergency room.

On the way we stopped to get our vehicle sprayed against the tsetse fly for we were now entering sleeping sickness coun-try. We were in luck. There were no roadblocks and no soldiers to be seen anywhere. Perhaps they all had a day off.

We arrived in Baluba in the late afternoon, as the sun was just beginning to dip beneath the western horizon. The convent was situated behind the hospital, almost on the shores of Lake Victoria, and already the two sisters living there were sitting out on the back veranda drinking tea and eating home-made scones. One was a small old sister from Donegal, Sr

Gracie, who had spent most of her life there and the other was a younger woman who later brought me around the hospital which was filled with patients suffering from TB, leprosy and sleeping sickness.

My weekend included Monday and all that time I just rested, read novels and enjoyed dosing in the sun, and listening to the stories of the good old days told in a quaint but attractive Donegal accent.

Kampala: 1983

Kampala itself was a city torn between various factions which were at one another's throats. And it was not a safe city.

Nightfall was always accompanied by the sound of gunfire. And on the nights when it was quiet we wondered whether the gunmen were taking a rest or merely preparing for a bigger assault the next night. Furthermore, we did not know who was fighting who and not even the locals could tell us. It all sounds bizarre now but at the time it was very real.

Since the public services had been disrupted, there was little or no street lighting, which made travel after nightfall extremely hazardous. However, daytime travel in the city was reasonably safe, especially for foreigners, although there were many instances of carjacking and even murder of expatriates, including priests and humanitarian workers in daylight hours.

Money was scarce and the shelves in the shops were almost empty. Yet the markets thrived and you could buy anything you wanted for a price.

Through all this the people kept their sense of hope, good humour and faith in the future. I saw too, how everyone helped his neighbour and, how people shared the little they had. I suppose it is easier to give when you have nothing to lose than give when you have a lot to lose.

Kampala Today

Today Kampala is a pulsating thriving city with luxury hotels and many imposing skyscrapers. Mulago is a huge hospital complex staffed by excellent nurses and doctors, and Makerere is once more a leading African University.

The people are as ebullient and unpredictable as ever, but they still retain the capacity to befriend the stranger and help the underdog as much as they did 40 years ago.

On my last visit in 2014, I travelled around on the back of a motorbike. This is the cheapest, quickest but also the most dangerous form of public transport in Kampala. You cling for dear life to the driver in front of you and must be ready to jump off instantly when danger looms. This can be a nightmare when negotiating a roundabout.

I had to jump off once on a particularly busy roundabout and my man drove off without me while I scampered to safety between buses, lorries, cars, donkeys, handcarts and bicycles. Traffic was very lawless that day and I needed all my wits about me to reach the safety of the footpath. My driver laughingly pulled up beside me a few minutes later and we continued our journey as if nothing amiss had happened.

An Honest Surprise

Had I not continued to use motorbike-taxis, I should not be able to tell the following story which says much for unexpected honesty.

On one occasion, the motorbike man charged me two dollars for a trip from my hotel to the city centre where I hoped to meet Dr Pius, one of my old Nsambya colleagues.

I had left my purse behind and I only had a twenty-dollar note in my pocket. So I gave it to him and, of course, he had no change. I should have guessed that he would have no change.

'Don't worry Sir', he reassured me, 'Just tell me where are you staying and I will return the change – eighteen dollars – tonight.' I hesitated but thought to myself 'What the hell, let him have a real bonus'. So I put the matter out of my mind – almost – but did tell him that I was staying at the Protea Hotel, a rather posh hotel where Mary Leader and Clive Lee, also from the College of Surgeons in Dublin, were staying.

That night came and went, so did the next night and so did several succeeding nights without me hearing or seeing anything of my eighteen dollars change. So imagine my amazement and delight when the barman came to me on the sixth night and handed me eighteen US dollars. I was stunned to find such honesty. I do not believe that I should have got my money back had this happened in New York, London or Dublin.

Kampala to Masaka

I have driven from Kampala to Masaka many times but, as is so often the case, one's first trip is the most memorable. Masaka lies about 130 kilometres southwest of Kampala on the west side of Lake Victoria, and while the journey takes about 90 minutes today, it took up to three hours in 1983 because of army check points and pot holes.

But it would take more than a war to deter traders for selling their wares on the roadside. Sometimes singly, but more often in groups, there were tables laden with fruit and yam and lots of stalls displaying the red Coca-Cola sign and many traders selling a variety of homemade furniture such as chairs tables and mattresses all at 'very special prices'.

I was especially taken by the typical Ugandan three-legged stool, which comes in both adult and child sizes. The design is simple, functional and elegant. Three short lengths of wood are bound together at 45° angles so that a circular bamboo seat can fit snugly into the concavity. Cleverly concealed nails hold the whole thing together, resulting in a sturdy portable little chair which is both practical and comfortable.

I later bought a few to give to friends at home but am now loath to part with them.

You will find a variety of stools in different parts of Africa. For example, in Ghana, there is the *ashanti stool*, in Angola, the *Budjok stool* and in the DCR, the *Buli stool*. Many of these are very ornate, but in my opinion none are as comfortable as the simple Ugandan three-legged one.

To reach Masaka, you must cross the equator, and this is a point where all visitors stop and take a mandatory photograph. It gives you a strange tingle to stand on the equator. There you are exactly half way between the North and South poles, with one foot in each hemisphere. Technically, you are like the Atlas, except that unlike him you are holding up the whole earth with your feet not with your head!

Even in the worst of times, there will be a persistent group of traders at the equator selling three-legged stools, juicy pineapples, bottles of doubtful water, packets of cigarettes and a *pot purri* of useless *bric a brac*. And they will run after you if you do not buy, or crowd around you, all vying for your attention. Dare leave your vehicle or they will physically press in on you and tug annoyingly at your sleeves in the process.

But the stop here is brief, we buy nothing, and quickly resume our journey further and further into the heart of Africa. Eventually, we reach Masaka.

Masaka is the second largest town in Uganda. It is not in any way a picturesque post-card town, but neither is it just a collection of hovels. There are many decent looking buildings in the main street and clearly this is a place of some importance. It is the administrative centre of the Masaka district and so plays an important role in the fabric of local life.

Like many important places in Africa, it has a long history of tribal violence, rebellions of one sort or another and of bloody massacres. Although it was quiet when I went there in 1983, it was the site of fierce clashes in the 1981–1986 Civil War when the fighting there sealed the exile of Milton Obote.

Ten years earlier, fighting in the region of Masaka was pivotal to the success of exiled Ugandans and Julius Nyerere's Tanzanian forces in ousting Idi Amin. The fighting at that time swayed from side to side until 1979 when the liberators finally 'thrashed Masaka' leaving Idi Amin no choice but to flee. Poor Masaka.

Kitovu Hospital

On my first visit, I saw little of the Masaka town. My destination was Kitovu Hospital which served the whole district. This hospital was started in 1955 and run by the MMMs until 2001 when it was handed over to the local authorities. It is now one of the foremost hospitals in Africa for treating VVFs.

The hospital itself lies on the summit of Kitovu hill and is reached by a narrow winding road which has hardly changed and certainly has not improved over the years. The location means that gentle breezes cool the wards at night but unfortunately at 1,300 metres it is not quite high enough to deter the mischievous mosquitoes that make a nightly feast on patients and staff alike.

Although now a State hospital, the MMM sisters still work there and the matron is an MMM sister. All the current MMMs in the hospital are African with the few remaining Irish ones living in two little bungalows at the back of the hospital proper but within the hospital compound. The Irish sisters do outreach clinics, mother and child clinics and HIV work. I have seen the transition from a totally expatriate administered hospital to one that is run by the Ugandans and it has been a happy and seamless handover. And one in which the standard of care continues to go up.

Sr Davnit from Ireland was the chief lab technician when I arrived. She was a small-sized nun who ran the lab with military precision. She was a born teacher for she even taught me how to do a Western Blot test – the latest technology. Shortly afterwards – cumbersome though it was – she used this test to diagnose HIV and this, no doubt, contributed greatly to focusing attention on the disease long before it was recognised in other places.

Sr Maura Lynch, another Irish sister, was the surgeon. Maura was an excellent surgeon and if I had time I could have learned a lot from her. Everyone who met Maura loved her and I was no exception. She is one of a long litany of wonderful women who gave their lives to serving others.

I also remember Helen Sharpe, from Donegal. She worked with local women teaching them basic hygiene and showing them how to prepare and use oral rehydration solution (ORS), which was then coming in vogue as a treatment for diarrhoea. Later she turned to working in AIDS programmes and, like Miriam Duggan in Nsambya, spent herself in helping the victims of this scourge which was starting to devastate Uganda.

In 1982, a year before I first arrived, the Sisters had received a container full of medical supplies, baby food and clothes. Once it was emptied they got the locals to partition it into several small sections. Openings for a door and window were cut into each section making each one an independent little room. In this way they managed to provide individual bedrooms for visitors like me.

Mostly I slept well in my terrace container room, but on other occasions, I hardly slept at all because of the din of pelting rain on the metal roof.

During the day we would take a break in a gazebo, a round structure like a bandstand, with stunning views of the countryside below. The sisters referred to this as their Portiuncula, after the little chapel near Assisi in Italy. Our gazebo was also used as a quiet place where one could pray or meditate or simply rest in spare moments during the day.

Recreation in the evening was always a happy time, a time that everyone looked forward to and during which everyone got a chance to talk about their day or write letters or exchange news from home. I suppose you could call it a family get-together.

If it were a Feast Day or someone's birthday then there were always special treats for everyone including drop-in visitors.

John Kelly

I have mentioned that Kitovu was a centre for repairing VVFs. This work had been pioneered by Ann Ward in Anua and one of her protégés there was John Kelly, an obstetrician from Birmingham, England. I met him for the first time many years later in Kitovu where, at the age of 80, he was still doing VVF repairs and showing his technique to surgeons from all over Africa and further afield.

I stayed with him in his little house and got to know him very well. In the evenings we chatted as only elderly men do, keeping back nothing and reminiscing about our medical experiences. He told me many stories about his time in Africa and more recently in Afghanistan, all of which were fascinating.

His personal life was without blemish. He practised austerity and self-discipline such as I have seldom encountered.

And he did so in such an unobtrusive and humble way that few were aware of his extraordinary spirituality. John too has passed away as have so many of my friends.

St Henrys

Not far from the hospital stood St Henrys, a thriving and prestigious boys school, founded in 1922 by Fr Laberge, a White Father and a protégé of the famous Cardinal Lavigerie. Woodcarving was a major trade taught there, and the boys turned out the most beautiful little figurines, statues and assorted objects, carved in teak, mahogany or bone. They also produced many boutique paintings depicting African village life or showing warriors in profile. I bought as many as I could afford but had my greedy eyes on one special painting of Christ on the cross. This was done in cubist style, similar to what Picasso might do, and I thought it was the most moving image of the suffering Christ I ever saw. I had not enough money to buy it but did eventually get it when I returned again to St Henrys some years later with my daughter Danielle. She hangs it proudly in her house in Dublin now. I have not been to St Henrys since but I have no doubt that it continues to turn out – not just fine art work – but excellent young men fully equipped to meet the needs of a modern Uganda.

Makondo

It was while I was in Kitovu that I made a weekend visit to Makondo. This was a very isolated little spot, well away from any main road, where there were really no modern facilities at all. The MMMs had a small house there and ran a primary Health Care Centre for the sick of the area. They bundled the very sick into their Land Rover and brought them to the

Kitovu Hospital. It was in Makondo that I first met Sr Dympna was a buxom, motherly, warm-hearted person always in good humour. She was a good golfer and bridge player yet, behind all her *bonhomie*, she had a practical and pragmatic nature.

Rabies

It was she who told me about rabies in the local population. The offending dogs had been slaughtered, but the fear of rabies had not disappeared because at the moment there were two people clearly stricken with the condition.

It was the first time I had seen rabies in humans and it was an experience I never wish to have again. Both were young men. They were very ill, too ill to move, and both died the day after I saw them. For the past few days, they had been hallucinating, acting violently and aggressively towards everyone and dribbling saliva continuously.

In some ways, they resembled patients with tetanus as their bodies arched in uncontrolled muscle spasms. But in addition, they screamed all the time, craved for water and went into wild convulsions at the sight of it, drooling animal like from their mouths.

The locals were afraid of them and so was I. The reason for our fear was not so much seeing them in torture or being afraid we would catch rabies if we touched them, but the awful terror that they would bite us. Human transmission of rabies has not been documented, but there were two cases I heard of later in Addis Ababa where everyone was certain that a rabid mother had transmitted rabies to her two children by biting them.

Both my patients were tied down which was the only way they could be controlled. I probably hastened death by giving morphia but their suffering was so intense that I would gladly have put them into a coma if I had the means.

Other than that I did no medical work in Makondo. I just rested in the afternoons and took leisurely walks in the mornings. Back in the convent in the evenings, I sat and talked with the sisters about Makondo and its problems. In particular, we talked about its isolation, the lack of basic needs and the health problems of the people.

My daughter Danielle and I visited Makondo some years later. This time we explored the vicinity of the convent more thoroughly than I had done when alone. One of our favourite walks was the rectangular route through the local countryside starting at the convent and ending exactly where we started. It is perhaps two miles in length and takes about 40 minutes to complete. The walk way is narrow, but two people can still stay abreast so that it is easy to make conversation. Stocky big-leafed banana trees, soaring palms, and tall rushes flank either side. Flowers abound, small and large, and flaunt their beauty uncaring whether men see them or not. Sometimes you come across a child scampering in the opposite direction. Sometimes there are a few huts off the track and sometimes a wart hog rushes beside you and dives into the undergrowth.

We used to love this walk absorbing the warmth, the colour and the sounds of deepest Africa. There was peace there.

It was here we really relaxed and I think that Danielle too was touched deeply by the experience.

I hold that all the wild uncultivated places of this earth are as much God's garden as the most artistic well-minded gardens of Versailles.

The Generator

In the evenings, we would sit around and chat – chat about nothing and about everything. I suppose having a seventeen-year-old girl with me brought a new dimension into the nuns' lives which, though challenging, were often dreary and monotonous. And for us it was nice too. Some of the serenity and gentleness of the Sisters rubbed off on us and drew us closer to God and nature.

Our light was provided by flickering Tilly lamps, which were blanketed with the dead bodies of mosquitoes and other flying insects.

They would often bemoan the fact that they had no generator. 'We could do so much more for these poor people if we had electricity' Dympna said. I wondered what they could do. 'We could deliver children at night, have decent lighting at all times, run a proper fridge instead of the old kerosene one we now use…Oh what a difference it would make'

'Have you any funds to put a deposit on one? …'No, mother house has no spare funds for that sort of thing … not for here anyway'

'What a shame… How much would you need?' Was I falling into a trap?

'Oh Lord….' She threw her eyes to heaven and then startled me by going to a drawer and pulling out a sheaf of official looking papers. 'Lets see…', she fumbled through the papers in her hand. 'To get what we want delivered here and fully installed would take ten thousand. Ten thousand sterling … That's way beyond anything we have or anything we can raise' she trailed off and we were all silent for a moment.

You know the way you automatically want to help anyone or support any worthwhile project that you really feel needs help. God, how I wished at that moment that I was a millionaire. But I had nothing like 10,000 pounds let alone a million. Yet something within me made me determined to get that generator. That something inside me – whether vanity or pride, I don't know – made me blurt out.

'I'll get you the ten thousand ... I'm sure I can raise it at home.' I trailed off, now a little hesitant. But I had gone beyond the point of no return. I regretted my foolhardiness almost immediately, but could not now retract. Ten thousand was then an enormous amount, more than I would earn in a year.

The sisters were ecstatic. I was their hero, their saviour. I was treated with extra special care and the local chief was informed of Dr Dom's promise.

All the time, inside me, I felt miserable, a fraud and a hypocrite. Mostly I knew I had been a big-mouthed fool. However, that was that. There was no going back. I put the whole affair out of my mind. I would think of it when I returned to Ireland. Meantime I continued to enjoy my R and R (rest and relaxation) in Makondo.

But I must come down to earth and tell you the end of the story of the generator and the ten thousands. The end of the story was unexpected. When I came home, I wrote to every agency I could think of looking for some part of the money I had promised. I hoped that I could make up the ten thousands by asking for smaller amounts from several sources rather than by asking for the whole lot together. All responded either negatively or not at all. I was especially disappointed in Trocaire, who had – in my view – become so non-denominational that they would not support projects which had – in their view – even a trace of a religious or proselytising mission.

This was nothing compared to my dismay when a letter that came telling me that the sisters had ordered a generator on the presumption that I could fund it. Well, yes, I had assured them I would come up good. They believed me – why wouldn't they – and since it would take so long between ordering the generator and its arrival in Makondo they had simply gone ahead and done so.

In desperation and, with little hope, I went to Dublin and called to the Head Office of the Allied Irish Bank, naively expecting to see the chief executive. I presented my name at the reception saying that I would only take a few minutes of his time and that it 'was a personal matter'.

The receptionist was more astonished than I when she got a reply from the chief executive's private secretary saying 'Mr Scanlon will see you right now.' I went up to a top floor and was led along a carpeted corridor finally arriving at a highly polished oak panelled door. On entering I was warmly welcomed by the boss himself.

He was Gerry Scanlon. Gerry had been in school in Newbridge with me and, although we were not close pals in those days (Gerry did not play rugby), we were always on good terms. Gerry was good at maths, better than me at 'figures'.

After school Gerry had joined the Bank and risen rapidly. He was efficient, astute in business, and certainly a leader. He listened to my request calmly and, without hesitation, wrote out a cheque there and then for 10,000 pounds. I was stunned and hardly able to express my thanks. I left with indecent haste and posted off the cheque immediately. I did not even have an account at the time in the AIB, although afterwards I opened one with them called *Peoplecare* into which I put any money given to me for charity.

Finally, there was a happy footnote to all this. I actually got the generator from Crusader Generators in the United Kingdom for £6,214 sterling. That meant that after exchange rates etc. we had money left over for the Health Centre in Makondo – a very welcome and unexpected bonus.

I found the original invoice recently in the bottom of a drawer.

By Bus from Kampala to Nairobi: 1984

Mariba Forest, Jinja, and the Nile

The Akamba bus has brought people from Kampala to Nairobi and back for many years. It crosses the border between Uganda and Kenya either at Busia or Kisumu. My bus was to cross at Busia. I was going home via Nairobi because flights from Entebbe were erratic and very expensive.

Our first stop was Lugazi, but we only remained there ten minutes or so which was just as well since my fellow travellers told me that it is hard to find anything of special interest in the town itself, although Lugazi is an important administrative centre. Shortly after leaving Lugazi, 25 miles east of Kampala, we entered the Mabira Forest.

The Mabira Forest teems with wildlife varying from exotic birds and mangabey monkeys to all kinds of insects and snakes. Fellow travellers on the bus told me that apes have attacked trucks and buses that stalled on their way through the forest, and to tell the truth, we all felt a little apprehensive when we saw inquisitive faces staring at us from nearby trees. Worse than apes is the danger of being attacked by bandits wielding machetés or AK-47s. So we were very relieved that the bus picked up speed as soon as it entered the dark menacing gloom where the overhanging branches of trees cut out the rapidly fading sunlight.

Jinja

Our bus passed through the forest unmolested and soon we arrived at Jinja, the last big town before reaching the border. We had now covered the 80 miles from Kampala in about two hours, which was exactly on schedule.

Jinja lies on the northern shore of Lake Victoria, just west of the White Nile, and for many years has been regarded as the source of that river. But this is disputed nowadays since some explorers have decided that the true origin is in Rwanda, where a small stream flows into Lake Victoria and then exits the lake at Jinja. Still others claim that the headwaters come from the Mountains of the Moon, specifically the Rwenzori range, in Uganda.

Whatever the truth there is always a sense of wonder when you visit the spot where Speke is alleged to have discovered the source of this great river, the longest river on earth. For it will continue from here all the way via Khartoum to break up into the Nile Delta which issues by hundreds of streams into the Mediterranean.

At Khartoum the White Nile joins the Blue Nile, which indisputably rises in Lake Tana, in the highlands of Ethiopia.

I pity the man whose heart does not beat faster the first time he beholds the confluence of these great rivers.

However, my heart was beating faster for another reason. It was time for us to disembark and face the ordeal of a border crossing at night hoping that we would not incur the displeasure of some petty official on either side.

We were now at the Busia border crossing, 68 miles beyond Jinja. There are two Busia towns, Busia Uganda and Busia Kenya, but it was dark and we could only see the dimly lit customs and immigration sheds on the Ugandan side. I follow the stream of people feeling a little out of place as the only white face among so many.

The actual crossing can be a seamless process or fraught with all kinds of danger from demands for money, to ceaseless rummaging in your bags, to answering endless, seemingly pointless questions (what is your mother's Christian name?) or sheer indifference where everyone, including those who push their way past you, gets attended except you.

Meantime it is hot and airless and you may even succumb to buying a dubious drink from one of the many vendors who press on you from every side. But have patience. There is order in all this apparent chaos, and eventually you will be seen and processed. And most of the time by friendly, polite but obviously bored officials.

As it happened, the officials hardly give me a glance but stamped my passport and chalked my luggage without a comment. I trudged a hundred yards or so after the crowd and repeated the whole procedure on the Kenyan side. It was one of the easiest border crossings I have ever made.

Our bus was waiting on the Kenyan side, one of many lined up across the road. The driver was standing at the door helping older people – and me – to climb aboard. It was good that I had noted the registration number of the bus, or otherwise I would have been going from bus to bus wondering which was mine and might well have been left behind.

I found my seat, pulled down the window blind and decided to try and sleep. I hardly noticed the lurch as the engines revved up and the bus resumed its journey to Nairobi.

It was morning when we pulled into the bus depot in Tom Mboya Street. There was much stretching and yawning but there was also a bounce in the step of the weary travellers who descended and stood singly and in little bunches breathing in the bracing Nairobi air. We were now in a peaceful city and felt elated at the prospect of going about our business freely and unhindered.

And yet, for the Ugandan travellers, and for me, this was a different country and we felt as all foreigners feel, just a bit out of things, on the outside looking in.

In time I became as comfortable in Kenya as I had been in Uganda. But that is another story.

Postscript

The Akamba bus company later became bankrupt and stood before the courts in Nairobi in 2012. For the best part of a century, it had provided safe and comfortable travel at affordable prices between Kampala and Nairobi. Other companies have since taken its place.

CHAPTER 10

THE ETHIOPIAN FAMINE, 1984–1985

Man's Part

This time it seemed that man was not responsible. This was no Biafra with armies clashing or no Cambodia with a mad regime imposing terror on its people. Yet the hand of man was there. In 1974, the seeds were already sown when an armed rebellion by the Marxist *Derg Movement* deposed the Emperor Haile Selassie.

The followers of Haile Selassie – and there were many worldwide – were known as Rastafarians. This name derives from his popular title in Ethiopia, *Ras Tafari* (prince Tafari). The adulation he received rested on the belief that Haile Selassi was the new Solomon, and indeed it seems that he really believed he was 'the anointed one' if not the incarnation of Solomon himself.

All that remains of his glory now are two stone lions at the entrance to his palace. He died while under house arrest in 1975, but the whereabouts of his body was a secret until his remains were discovered in 1992 – buried under a toilet in the Imperial Palace. You can see his present resting place in Trinity Cathedral in Addis Ababa where he was finally interred in the year 2000. A sad end for the Lion of Judah.

Haile Selassie, initially a strong and farseeing ruler, had become a tyrant by 1974. He watched, seeming unmoved, as his people died in their hundreds of thousands from famine and disease.

No wonder the *Derg Movement* had the support of the people, at least initially. But very quickly the people became disillusioned and the subsequent devastation of people's lives and of the countries' economy made fertile ground for the growth of yet another group, the *Red Regime*, headed by Comrade Mengistu.

Mengistu was a ruthless man with little time for the niceties of life or the rights of individuals. From 1977 onwards, he ruthlessly exploited the population with land confiscation, widespread imprisonments and multiple assassinations. As seems the usual tale in Africa, the rule of Mengistu – as of the *Derg* and Haile Selassie before him – ended in bloodshed. By 1991 he was overthrown and the Ethiopian People's Revolutionary Democratic Front (EPRDF) seized power.

There were many 'little famines' throughout these turbulent years but the 'great famine', precipitated by an unprecedented drought and continuous fighting, did not strike the land until 1983.

In that year the economy of Ethiopia was in ruins. Mengistu was in power and, while he and his colleagues lived off the fat of the land, the ordinary Ethiopian was either starving or barely surviving at subsistence level. The world was losing patience but did not intervene apart from mouthing the usual pious platitudes.

Nature's Part

Even Mother Nature had lost patience and decided to teach Man a lesson. She now intervened perversely by further punishing the innocent people of Ethiopia and Eritrea. She let the land bake and allowed a scorching sun to the burn the already arid earth. She even mocked us by sending rain-filled clouds scudding across the high blue skies, only to disappear slowly over the horizon.

Invocations, rain dances, prayers and sacrifices of appeasement to guarding spirits were all in vain. Day by day the anguish of the upturned haggard faces worsened, and day-by-day bodies became weaker and more emaciated. Wells dried up, little rivers disappeared and big rivers became muddy pools. This was now a country that was becoming a living hell. And the world waited, indifferent and uninformed. First the crops failed. Then cattle, sheep and goats died, and, finally, the hot wind scattered their desiccated bones over the unforgiving dusty landscape.

Soon it was the turn of the humans to die. Initially old men and old women died, and then anyone whose health was already less than 100 per cent succumbed. Finally, starvation and disease claimed the lives of men, women and children of all ages.

Wild animals did best, scavenging on the dead carcasses of anything they could find. And they scavenged human bodies, even so far as mauling and eating children who were still alive.

The World Listens at Last

If the world stirred to the plight of those caught up in the Biafran War of the 1960s, it sat up sharply when pictures of the Ethiopian famine came on the TV screens in the 1980s. The early reporting by Michael Buerk, and the exclusive pictures he showed us of children dying of starvation, was the tinderbox that ignited the world's conscience to the unfolding disaster that was striking so many innocent people.

Thousands of hunger-stricken families trekked long distances to find pasture for the few animals that survived and, when none was found, and they had eaten their last meal, they walked mile after mile searching for something, anything, to eat. Every mile they went cost one or more lives when those unable to go further simply curled up on the side of the road and waited for a blessed release from this life.

To me there seemed to be two sorts of reaction by people in these extreme stages. One was complete lethargy where the person was listless, disinterested, simply a living dead, a zombie. Others showed restlessness, had quick darting eyes, fidgeted with their clothes and held their hands out appealingly – not for money – but for food.

Often the nights were cold and people simply died of hypothermia. Sometimes their blood sugar would go so low that they died of hypoglycemia. In most cases, death was hastened by overwhelming diarrhea, cholera, typhus and other infections. Children were among the most vulnerable, and both measles and meningitis were added nightmares in their case.

Makele Camp

I worked with the International Committee of the Red Cross (ICRC) in a large camp just outside the town of Makele. The camp itself housed about 100,000 people but my chief responsibility was the care of children. Officially, we handled over 1,000 children in special feeding programmes and managed 50 of the worst – including the sick ones – in a special nutrition tent. Unofficially I am certain we dealt with many more.

For those of you who have never been to a refugee camp let me describe the one in Makele. At ground level, it may have looked like a disorganised sea of white tents. But from the air you realised that the tents were all nicely spaced and had clear passages between them. Furthermore, the whole camp was divided into discrete numbered sectors or *arrondissements*, which were autonomous; little communities in themselves. Water trucks came intermittently to each sector and the people would fill any receptacle they could with clean drinking water, which was more valuable than liquid gold. Containers varied from small buckets, empty coke cans and coconut shells to sophisticated water canisters. I even saw a child trying vainly to fill a rubber balloon with water. Food was also delivered so that the people could make their own *injera* or boil rice and fry fish according to their own tastes. Food supplies were limited but we did our best to provide an average of up to 2,000 calories per day to each person. In many sectors, everyone went to a communal kitchen where food was prepared and doled out to them ensuring fairness as much as possible.

Initially we sunk several deep wells on the site. But these became a liability for water was wasted as it splashed everywhere and worse still any remaining pools of water became perfect breeding spots for mosquitoes. We did try to reduce this waste by replacing the taps with pressure activated ones that automatically closed off when not in use. At least this stopped the dreadful waste of water the occurred when ordinary taps were left running all night.

These spring-controlled taps were difficult to source – I don't know why – and even the engineers had great difficulty in getting them. But when we got them we reduced water loss dramatically.

Waste disposal is a problem everywhere and no more so than in a refugee camp. However, we were concerned only with human body waste for there was virtually no other waste in the camp. So we got the people to dig deep trenches, which would serve as communal latrines. We paid a small fee to designated refugees to pour lime into them each evening, and we also employed 'latrine watchers' to make sure that the latrines were used in an orderly and appropriate manner. People vied with one another to get these jobs which were an important source of income for the lucky ones.

To use the toilet you crouched astride the trench and did your business as best you could without slipping in. However some did fall in, especially children. And that was not a pleasant sight. Unfortunately, we had no facility for those who used the latrines to wash their hands or clean themselves afterwards. However, we did erect corrugated sheet fencing on both sides of the trench so that some semblance of privacy could be maintained, especially for the women.

There was little privacy for those short-taken however. For many, the diarrhea was so severe that there was no time to get to the latrine before nature called. Makele Camp was the only place I have ever been where I regularly saw men and women defecate beside each other without shame or embarrassment. This gives you some idea of the loss of personal dignity people endured, but strangely, I saw no shame in it, was not embarrassed by it, and merely passed by, accepting such scenes as unfortunate but unavoidable and indeed *normal* under the circumstances.

There was also a delousing area into which recently arrived refugees were led. Here they were stripped naked, washed, deloused and de-scabied by painting them with benzyl benzoate or gentian violet. Scabies was almost universal. The condition is very contagious and spreads like wildfire in crowded unsanitary conditions where people are huddled together and clothes are not washed. It was simply another plague on top of the pre-existing misery that people had to suffer. The scratching is constant, the itch almost unendurable at night, and once again it tests all your faith in a merciful Almighty to accept it as either fair or just or reasonable.

Lice, ticks, mites, snakes, spiders, scorpions, hungry hyenas and the ubiquitous mosquito now became very important to me. One becomes very earthy when working in a refugee camp. Trying to preserve the norms of civilised society soon becomes superfluous and then irrelevant.

Law and order does not come naturally to any large group of people and without the presence of a well-disciplined detachment of the Ethiopian army there would have been chaos. Every morning hundreds, sometimes thousands of people, waited at the entrance to the camp begging for admission. We did our best to accommodate everyone but would have been quite unable to control the flow of refugees to manageable proportions were it not for the soldiers who guarded the front gates.

Other soldiers patrolled the perimeter, which was a job that might normally have been done by hired watchmen. All this gave a sense of security to those inside and as a result things were amazingly orderly.

While I was there, the number of refugees reaching our camp increased daily. Most of them were covered in nothing more than a dull shapeless brown cloak made out of the coarse sacking in which donated maize and rice had been carried. They came silently in a never-ending flow, like some sort of biblical trek from the *Old Testament*.

TV never catches the fullness of grief when reporting these scenes. It cannot catch the sadness in the way people shuffle along, it cannot transmit the pleading in the peoples' eyes, it cannot immerse you in the atmosphere of grief, hopelessness and desperation that fills the very air you breath as you see, smell and feel the suffering of so many pathetic human beings.

Cholera

On entering through the main gates you faced a broad pathway that roughly divided the camp into two.

My place of work was immediately to the left of the main gate but the cholera tent, also on the left, was at the far end of the dividing road and stood apart not just by its position but also by being somewhat larger than the other tents. It was here that we rehydrated our cholera patients.

Unless a patient could walk, he or she was carried to the tent on a simple canvas stretcher, which we laid lengthways across two wooden supporting blocks, each about 3 feet high and 3 feet wide. The wooden side poles could then be slipped out, leaving the patient lie on the canvas, with his head and shoulders supported by one block and his legs by the other. The poles were then used to complete a stretcher for the next patient.

A hole had been cut in the centre of the canvas so that the patient could defecate directly into a bucket or into a black plastic bag placed beneath. The volumes of feces passed in cholera can be enormous. It is just like turning on a tap.

I attended adults as well as children, although children were my main concern. Among the adults I recall one in particular, probably because the way I treated him does not do me much credit.

This young man came into my clinic one morning looking well but complaining of acute pain in his calves. On questioning he admitted to passing loose stools during the previous twelve hours.

The two things seem unrelated at first glance, but I should have been immediately aware of the linkage between cholera and calf pain. In the massive diarrhea of cholera – as in any 'secretory' diarrhea – the volume of fluid lost is so great that the body becomes rapidly depleted of salt. This loss of salt, particularly of potassium salt, causes muscle cramps, which can be very severe. Whatever the scientific reason, I should have known that pain in the calf together with diarrhea is a red light. Urgent rehydration is needed.

Instead I prevaricated. Yes, I admitted him to the cholera unit but no, I did not refuse his request that he might go home – he was a local from Makele – and inform his family. He promised he would be back in a couple of hours and I agreed.

He was carried into the camp at about 4 p.m. that afternoon and, despite receiving massive infusions of fluid intravenously, he died at 6 p.m. the same day.

You move on from these situations but every time they happen, you learn a bit more and, I hope, you become a better doctor.

Examine the Patient Not the Notes

My immediate predecessor here was a Swiss doctor, Pierre Peron. He was an excellent doctor. Precise, conscientious and caring. He was especially excellent in documenting everything and certainly I was no match for him in that regard. At that time Irish doctors were very lax in recording notes about patients and, when they did write something, it was probably illegible. This has changed and Irish doctors and nurses now follow the standards long in use in North America and mainland Europe. I expect the threat of litigation has been the main spur.

Unfortunately nowadays the medical profession may spend more time writing about patients than in examining them. I once accompanied a senior doctor on ward rounds in the Mayo Clinic in Rochester, Minnesota. He barely noticed the patient. He consulted the notes, which were beautifully displayed on a monitor over the bed, after which he turned to his accompanying entourage and got briefed on things like 'How did the patient sleep last night?' and 'Is there much pain now?' … 'What are home conditions like?' I wondered; 'Why not ask the patient directly?'

He then took questions from the most eager of his retinue about the actual 'Disease' in the bed, before moving on and saying 'Let's take a look at the prostate cancer in the next bed!'

In truth I have also been guilty of this sort of thing. I can recall saying to medical students 'there is a lovely spleen down in bed five…you ought to go and examine the mitral stenosis in ward six if you want to hear a real diastolic murmur.' I hope I have learned a little over the years.

Now I say to students 'Listen to the patient carefully he will tell you the diagnosis from his own lips in more than 80 per cent of cases and if you cannot diagnose a fractured wrist or broken hip without an MRI or PEP scan, you have no business being a doctor.'

The Children's Unit

My own unit nominally held 50 sick children. On many occasions, we had double that number but somehow we managed.

We housed them in a large rectangular tent fitted with plastic windows and in which small beds and cots were lined up in four rows, one along each wall and two in the centre, back to back. There was an extension towards the end where we could treat emergencies and in which the doctor and nurses kept records. The nurses were a mixture of Swiss volunteers and locals and the ward clerk was a handsome and very helpful Ethiopian man.

Severe dehydration from gastroenteritis, with vomiting and diarrhea, was the major cause of death in our Unit. Dehydration also followed measles and other infectious diseases, but in virtually all cases the child's defences were already lowered by a lack of food.

Day after day, we were inundated by a flood of infants and children all needing immediate rehydration and, as often as not, we could not cope. The simple fact was that we could not physically manage to set up IV infusions on every one. Many of these little ones were already moribund but that simply made their treatment a matter of greater urgency. Nowadays, one might possibly handle such children by giving fluids directly into the tibia, the major bone of the leg below the knee. I was not then familiar with this technique although I had heard it was a very simple one.

So my immediate problem remained. How could I get a dying child – who could no longer swallow – sufficiently hydrated, so that the collapsed veins would fill and a conventional IV line could be set up. I had tried giving fluids by the intraperitoneal route a few years earlier, and had been impressed by how easy it was to push a needle into the abdomen and deliver fluid that way. So we introduced the technique here in Makele.

This proved a quick and easy way of priming the circulatory system and it certainly worked on some children and possibly saved a small number of lives.

The nurses quickly learned the technique and became more adept than I. Ultimately, working as a team, we could set up infusions on twenty children in urgent need of fluids within ten minutes.

Occasionally, when a baby was moribund and grossly dehydrated, I would set up an IV via the jugular vein in the neck. This method could deliver a large amount of fluid rapidly and I normally held the child steady in my arms during the procedure. But I do not think I saved a single child that way. Indeed it may be that this intimate contact with lice infested children was the cause of an illness that almost killed me.

The mothers were grateful for anything we did, even if the child died. In most cases the child survived and, before discharge, the local staff would demonstrate how to make and administer ORS. ORS has proved to be the most important single advance in saving lives in developing countries in my lifetime.

Night Rounds

I worked as hard as I could, either doing clinics or working in the ward from early morning until evening. My night round finished the day. That was at 9 p.m. I always find 'night rounds' a real pleasure. Patients are mostly asleep or, if awake, you can give a smile or word of encouragement as you pass by. Children make their own funny noises, sometimes snorting, sometimes sighing and sometimes just breathing heavily. The evening light is kinder to everything and the nurses are generally in better form and less stressed than during the mad rush of day.

I have found the same of thing when working in hospitals at home and perhaps that is why some nurses prefer permanent night duty to working normal daylight hours.

Our Red Cross group stayed in a 'hotel' not far from the camp. It stood on a hill and was probably quite an elegant place in its day. It was a stone building on which the original white paint was now a streaky brown and was desquamating like the rash in scarlet fever. The hotel owners were delighted to have us. We brought welcome dollars, spent liberally and treated everyone with courtesy and respect. Our group was made up of French and Swiss volunteers apart from one English girl, Elizabeth Twitch and one Irish man (me). So we spoke French all the time and, although I had opted for Greek instead of French in school, I gradually picked up enough French to carry on a limited conversation.

I was lucky in that I had a room to myself, at the very top of the building, and so I not only had privacy but also had fewer mosquito visitors at night than anyone else. This relative isolation was soon to serve me badly but at the time I was delighted with my little retreat in the garret.

A Special Nun

When I wasn't working I either rested or read. It was easier to read a book that I had enjoyed previously so I re-read *The Lord of the Rings*. In the late afternoon there might be a jeep available and I would drive to Mass in a local church or visit other Aid Agencies. One afternoon I got a chance to visit a health centre where I was told 'an energetic Irish nun runs the show... has been working there for years.' I found the place easily enough. It was a little outside the town, a small wooden building shaded by large eucalyptus trees.

There were flowers outside, carefully tended and watered. Clearly the hand of the Irish nun was not confined to just tending the sick. But she was not expecting me and I was not sure how welcome another 'medical tourist' would be. I need not have worried. The door was opened by a tall thin white lady in a grey plaid skirt and short sleeved white blouse. She looked anything but a nun, well not my stereotype nun in a long habit, black veil, white coif and white apron. However, she did have a small religious symbol pinned to her blouse, perhaps a cross, I am not sure.

She welcomed me warmly and guided me into a small waiting room where she made me feel immediately 'at home'. She told me she was Margaret, Sr Margaret, a member of the English branch of the Daughters of Charity '... and had come out here to provide health care to the locals...Oh... quite unrelated to the famine...at first.' She emphasised 'at first'.

She then went on to explain that a most important aim of the Health Centre was to diagnose, treat and prevent trachoma at an early stage, before irreparable damage had been done to the person's eyesight. This was relatively easy. All that was needed was to teach people to wash their hands often, to shield their eyes against dust and not to rub them incessantly once they became infected or irritated. The next stage was to use tetracycline eye ointment, which was wonderfully effective in killing the causative bacterium, *Chlamydia trachomatis*. This was ludicrously inexpensive. Each tube of tetracycline only cost a few cents. But to be effective it had to be used early on in the disease and the patient had to be taught *and practise* decent hygiene. Not easy where there was no water.

The third stage was to do an operation, under local anaesthesia, to repair eyelids that had turned in on themselves (entropion). Turned in eyelids allow the eyelashes to irritate and scratch the already damaged cornea. As a result, there is scarring and vision becomes blurred through the thickened sclerotic cornea. Ultimately, the cornea becomes opaque and complete blindness results. The surgeon who did this operation in Makele was in fact herself.

Margaret showed me her technique and, after doing it a few times, I found that I could manage it quite well, if not as deftly as she.

On hearing that I was from Galway she asked if I knew her sister, Sabina, the wife of Michael D Higgins, who later became a distinguished President of Ireland. Galway is a small place and of course I had met 'Michael D' and Sabina. Afterwards, they told me how proud they were of that remarkable woman.

Sr Margaret is now back in her head convent in the United Kingdom, presumably to retire. She is just one of the many unsung heroines of our times.

Important Visitors

The Ethiopian famine was like a magnet for important people, including well-known journalists, politicians, movie stars and other celebrities. They came from the 'outside' world to see the famine with their own eyes. They would then fund-raise at home to support our efforts. To do this they appeared on TV chat shows, lobbied politicians and addressed public meetings in their home countries. They could speak authentically of the terrible sufferings they had seen in the camps, and mobilise millions of 'ordinary' people to come to our aid, by holding big charity concerts or by hosting special 'giving days' on TV. Bob Geldof was probably the most notable mobiliser of public donations and his name will forever be linked with Band Aid and the best-selling record *Do They Know It's Christmas?*

I did not want to spend precious time escorting such notables around, but many others were more than willing, and that did not bother me. However I did meet Diana Ross, the American singer, and nearly met Cardinal Basil Hume of Westminster. Both were genuinely moved by the distress all around them. I also spent a moment with Harry Belafonte, the West Indian singer, who will always be associated in my mind with the song *This is My Island in the Sun*.

I was told afterwards that he donated a cheque for a million dollars.

So Harry, you will not remember me, but I remember you, and will never forget your generosity.

Those of us who have worked in disaster situations are ambivalent about visits from celebrities especially from politicians.

We are perhaps envious of the publicity they get while we slog away – unnoticed Cinderellas. We often think – and surely unfairly in many cases – that they have ulterior motives in making these grand public gestures. Do they really care? They travel first class, they stay in the best hotels, they are usually protected by their own and by local security men, they eat well, they then hold a dying child, smile into TV cameras and ask ordinary people at home to donate as much as they can.

We are also aware that they drive around in fine sedans while we bump along in rickety old jeeps – if we are lucky. It is all so choreographed that it is hard not to be cynical.

Yet if all the money raised were well spent it would be difficult to complain. But this is not so. Who knows in the end how much of every dollar or euro raised is spent wisely? Certainly I don't.

Sixty Per Cent

My previous experience in the Biafran famine had taught me much about categorising malnutrition and starvation. Thus I was familiar with quick assessment techniques of a child's nutritional status and would grade them out of 100. There are many simple ways of doing this which take into account age, sex and race. Most are based on standard wt./ht. charts, abdominal girth or upper arm thickness. I remember that in Biafra the Quaker team had devised a simple stick, which I called the 'quakerstick', against which the child stood and you simply read off a figure indicating the child's nutritional status. We also had a formula from which we could tell how much milk and how many calories per day were needed so that we could start the optimum feeding programme.

The malnourished child is unable to fight infection normally and can easily die from diarrhea, measles or a chest infection. There is also the danger of dying from hypothermia or a low blood sugar and although we tried to avoid both of these but I do not know how successful we were.

However one fact became obvious early on. The mortality rate among those children who had lost over 60 per cent of their standard body weight was virtually 100 per cent and the mortality rate of those between 50 and 60 per cent weight loss was only somewhat less.

This fact became suddenly of crucial importance when it was discovered that the camp had only two weeks food left to feed everybody.

A hard decision needed to be made. Higher authorities flew in from Europe and conferred with the camp managers and I assume with the ICRC delegate and the various Program Directors of the different NGOs working in Makele.

I was completely oblivious to all this until I heard one night that from now on we should refuse entry to the Camp to those who were 60 per cent or more malnourished. The simple logic was that food was running out and it was clear that the under 60 per cent cohort had zero chance of survival.

I knew it made sense; it was a logical although not an easy decision to make. We could save so many more people if we conserved what we had for those with a chance of survival.

This was the message I got around the dinner table that night and it made my blood boil. I sometimes wonder whether I am dreaming all this but then I remember vividly what happened next day.

I arrived around 7.30 a.m. to the Camp. There was the usual crowd of people waiting outside the gate hoping to be admitted. They all looked miserable, they all looked exhausted and they all stood there silently, just waiting and hoping. Two armed soldiers stood at the Camp entrance and it was clear that no one could enter without their permission.

I took in the scene and saw a very thin emaciated boy, half standing, half leaning against an adult, almost directly opposite the Camp entrance. I knew immediately that he was not long for this world. Anyone would know, just one look at that tired little face and emaciated body would tell you that he had enough, and could go no further.

I scooped him into my arms, and marched straight into the Camp between the two soldiers who guarded the main entrance. They let me pass without a word. I walked slowly up the main passage between the rows of tents where the people now stopped doing whatever they were at and looked at this strange spectacle. In my arms was a tall lad, someone who would have probably been a great long distance runner or basketball player, but not any more. A deep silence descended on the place. I was conscious of the hush, but kept on going.

A young Ethiopian camp orderly joined me after a few moments and the three of us went to the last tent on the row, which was actually empty, ready for a new family. I sat down on something. I suppose it was a stool. I can't remember. I cradled the boy's head in my arms and he opened his eyes and gazed at me for a moment.

I took a jelly sweet from my pocket and placed it on his tongue. I imagined he smiled. Definitely he made some sort of effort to say thanks. And then he died. There and then.

I cannot recall this episode without reliving deep emotions of sadness, tears and anger at a world that can allow such things to happen.

The following day I was called to the office of the local Commandant. This was a command not an invitation. His office was situated on the other side of town and, as we passed through the market place, I could see sacks of rice for sale clearly labelled 'Gift from the people of the USA'. It was obvious to anyone that much of the relief aid from the outside world was falling into the hands of black marketeers and used for their profit rather than for the relief of the starving. Indeed the market was a thriving hub of selling and buying where you could get anything you wanted if you had money.

However, my thoughts were not on the rights and wrongs of things but on my own predicament. I had settled on the opinion that I would be deported, but was sure it would be a nice civilised deportation and that I would not be jailed. I was quite unrepentant for breaking the 60 per cent rule and, for once, I seemed to have the courage to defy authority irrespective of the consequences.

In a short time, we reached our destination which was a low white building approached by a central avenue. Several army vehicles were parked on the sun-yellowed grass on either side of the path, and several soldiers with carelessly slung rifles lounged about.

However, they suddenly came to life when our jeep drove up to the front door of the main building. My appearance was clearly a welcome break from the normal routine.

There were guards on either side of the door but they had obviously been expecting me for they let me in without even asking who I was, while the driver returned to the jeep. A lady, dressed in civilian clothes, greeted me formally in the hallway and said the Commandant would see me presently.

I took the seat she indicated and then she went behind her desk and continued reading a magazine. I settled for a long wait. That is the way of bureaucracy in most countries and in particular in developing countries. You spend hours and hours waiting in offices for someone to attend to you and when they do, they move slowly and languorously, as if they were sleep walking. Yet ultimately things get done.

Unfortunately, more often than not, you are asked to come back tomorrow and that is a bad sign. Because tomorrow may be a holiday, or a Friday (in Muslim countries) or a Saturday/Sunday (in Christian countries) or all these days in many countries. More often than not the person who deals with your affairs is not 'on seat', he is at a meeting or has been called away.

Westerners get very uptight about the slow pace by which their business is transacted in these situations. But that is counterproductive. Often the more the Westerner gets frustrated and shows signs of irritability the slower will he get his business done. It is better to be patient, to treat everyone with courtesy and to be prepared to sit and sit and sit – and smile at everyone. Eventually they will attend to you if only to get rid of you from the office.

However, I had only a wait of five minutes before a door facing the main entrance opened, and a smartly dressed officer called my name and beckoned me to follow him. He stood aside as I entered a large bright room with full-length windows and, opposite me, two large glass doors opening on to a private patio. It took me a few moments to make out the large figure of the Commandant who faced me with his back to the glass doors and his elbows resting on a huge mahogany table on which the sole object was an ancient black bakelite telephone.

This meant that while I was lit up by the sunshine the man at the desk scrutinising me was in shade. He was brief and to the point.

'Dr Colbert, please sit down'

I obeyed and waited for more.

'I have been informed that there is a shortage of food in the Camp outside town'

'We have only two weeks food left ... and we are receiving more and more people every day' and then unnecessarily I added, 'It's my duty as a doctor to help everyone no matter how near death....'

He held up his hand and said 'I am not here to discuss that Doctor....'

I really felt put down now but at least I had made my point. I muttered something about having now only enough food to give 1,400 calories per day to adults. Not half enough for their needs. But he was not interested. Then came the bombshell.

'Ah, doctor, you are in luck. We have two warehouses full of food that you can access. But for technical and administrative reasons only my men can issue the food to you and it will be in fixed amounts each day.' He shifted his chair and added 'And only for this emergency mind'.

I was astonished and thrilled.

My eyes had become accustomed to the glaring light and I could now see the shining medals on his chest and the red shoulder epaulets from which hung short tresses of thin golden cords. All these decorations were backdropped by his spotless camouflage tunic so that he looked a very smart Commandant indeed.

When he stood up to dismiss me I put out my hand and he grasped it firmly. Then he wished me good luck and I departed walking on air.

We used to say 'How come Mengistu is so fat and all the other Ethiopians are so thin?' It was of course a derogatory statement implying that Mengistu and his clique lived off the fat of the land while everyone else starved. But here was one fat Commandant or Commissar who was fat *and good*. I do not know who that man was, but he probably did more to save lives than anyone else I came across while in Makele.

Of course, we knew the army took whatever they wanted from the aid cargoes that landed in the airport. We had seen this with our own eyes. But to open two whole warehouses full of food so that we could feed the hungry was something beyond our wildest dreams.

An Air Drop

Before leaving the topic of food supplies I should mention that getting food to remote areas is always a problem. The dreadful roads, the lack of transport, the distances involved and the sometimes atrocious weather make delivering aid to everyone in need very difficult. And so it was decided to use airdrops as an alternative.

We were informed that an airdrop was to take place on a certain afternoon in a certain location and, since I had never seen an airdrop, I was anxious to go along and observe one. It meant skipping an afternoon's work but I felt it was worth it. Besides, the nurses, both Ethiopian and expatriate, were very capable of doing most – if not all – of the things I did.

Luckily the afternoon was calm and fine (actually every afternoon was calm and fine) so conditions were perfect for an airdrop. We chugged out of Makele, up a mountain track and eventually stopped in a high valley where the Army had posted roadblocks.

It was a perfect vantage point to see the giant Hercules come in, right on schedule. It swooped low enough for us to see the pilot and then he made a gentle curved ascent while the back of the plane opened and discharged its contents like some monster disgorging its prey. The food parcels sailed serenely to the ground like scattered confetti and even as the plane banked sharply to make another run people appeared as if from nowhere and started running to pick up the parcels. I am sure the pilot saw them but anyway he made another run and spilled out lots more parcels. Then he disappeared over the crest of the mountain and made his way back to Addis.

Many of the parcels burst open in mid-air, many got destroyed on impact with the ground and many were scattered over a wide area. However, the whole spectacle was fascinating and while the exercise may not have been cost-effective, it certainly must have provided food for many who would otherwise go hungry.

Hunger was not in evidence at a party the Italians NGOs gave on the Friday night following the air drop. I was not feeling well for a few days and, since I had a fever, I suspected malaria. I immediately started antimalarial tablets and paracetamol, but something inside me told me this was not malaria. As a precaution I added Septrin, an excellent drug in a variety of infectious conditions. Surely this would do the trick. Besides, it was the only antibiotic I had in my suitcase.

At this point I was sure that I had nothing serious. So on Friday night I went happily to a party in the 'Italian house'. I arrived at about six o'clock and drank a beer with Don Caesare, the very popular Italian priest who did the work of two men in the camps. Don Caesare was a big fat man, always laughing, and he spoke English exactly as you expect Italians to speak English. For the entire world he was the embodiment of the fictional Don Camillo, and I told him so.

He laughed, swigged his bottle and grinned.

'Dére be a bigga de difference ... Don Camillo talka de crocifisso, and de Lord, Him answer him ... but me ... not nobody hear me'

He was wrong. I reminded him that he spoke so loudly that everyone in the place could hear him. He bellowed laughing and shook his head saying 'You Irish...plenty too much ... plenty too much....'

I then told him I was not feeling well and would leave early to check on the sick children. So he saw me off at about eight o'clock and I made my way on foot to see my charges.

My fever must have heightened my senses for I remember everything quite vividly about that night. I clearly remember doing my rounds, talking to the nurse, checking on the sicker children and saying *bon soir* to all and then walking home.

It was a beautiful night, the sky a dome of purple, studded with stars that glittered and glimmered in their own mysterious worlds. Down here, on earth, the air was warm and humid but the oppressive heat of the afternoon was gone and an atmosphere of peace had descended like an invisible cloak that hid all the eyesores of the day. I climbed the rickety stairs to my garret and now felt a wave of weariness descend on me like a blanket. I was too tired to undress. I fell asleep and entered a world of dreams, fantasies and nightmares.

Typhus, A Disease of Dirt

I woke up while it was still dark with a blinding frontal headache. I took another gram of paracetamol but it brought no relief. And now I started getting stomach cramps and spent the rest of the night in and out of the bathroom with retching, vomiting and diarrhea. Towards dawn I was reduced to crawling to the toilet. I now had no toilet paper or any means to wash my hands. I was a mess. An embarrassed, useless mess.

Next morning was Saturday and I was unable to get up but my staff had previously told me to take Saturday and Sunday off to rest and so no one missed me. Saturday merged with Sunday and I gradually became comatose.

It was Tuesday before anyone came to see me. Strangely enough my visitor – I am told – was a 'nun' who had worried about my absence from Mass on Sunday and got a premonition that something was amiss with me. By Tuesday she could wait no longer but came in person to our lodging, climbed up the steep stairs and entered my room. She saw at once that I was very ill.

I know that there was a great hullaballoo after this and I know that Dr John Good, an Irish doctor, came to see me and insisted I be evacuated immediately. I have no recollection of how they carried me down the rickety hotel stairs and that must have been quite a job. But I have some memory of being lifted into the back of an ambulance outside. It remains in my memory as a time freeze in which everything is instantaneously clear but in which events before and after are completely blotted out.

I have no recollection of being put on a plane but I was told afterwards that they flew me to Asmara a distance of over 1,500 km by road but only 200 km by air and I do not know whether we refuelled there or whether I was transferred to another plane.

However, I do remember something very painful happened to me at some stage during that flight. It seems the nurse they had sent out from Geneva to mind me on the flight could not pass a normal rubber catheter into my bladder and resorted to using a metal one. Seeing me in a coma and, probably believing that I could feel no pain, he went ahead. Believe me that this is about the most painful thing that can happen to a man. He must have pushed it in very roughly as I still recall some fleeting moments of excruciating deep-seated pain during that trip. The pain must have lightened my coma for during it I was conscious of the drone of the engines. I knew I was in an aeroplane.

At odd moments too I was dimly conscious of the shape of a person near me, presumably the nurse. I actually think he did a sort of prostatectomy or perhaps tunnelled out a false passage to my bladder, as I understand there was a lot of bleeding at the time. It mattered little; the end result was they could now monitor my urinary output.

All this had one unexpected dividend. Unlike most of my contemporaries, I have never had any prostate trouble since!

On a more serious note it taught me that even though you think someone in a coma can feel no pain, and even if he or she makes no visible response to a painful stimulus, nurses and doctors should always treat such a person with respect and care in what they say within earshot and in what they do such as passing a catheter or setting an IV or passing a stomach tube. Never assume a comatose patient is an inert unfeeling 'object'.

I know now that our final destination was London. Unfortunately, we were barely ten minutes left Asmara when my heartbeat became irregular and my blood pressure started to fall. The pilot was advised to divert to Geneva rather than go the extra miles to London. Meantime, my nurse kept an IV going and hoped for the best. I do not remember landing in Geneva airport but do remember being pushed on a trolley into the emergency department of the Cantonal University Hospital.

As I crossed the portals my heart went into VFib (ventricular fibrillation). However the cardiac arrest team was there, waiting for me and, for sure, I should have died otherwise.

Out-of-Body Experience

I hesitate to write about this. Many others have had a similar experience and people are tired listening to and reading the same old descriptions. However the truth is that people who have had an out-of-body experience *always want to talk about it* and I am no exception. So here goes.

While the medics were working on me, quite suddenly, I was conscious that some inner part of me was starting to leave my body. It was as if a photograph of my whole self was rising in the air, a transparent photograph without substance or weight or any physical attribute that could be grasped or felt. I could see both above me and below me *at the same time*, and this did not feel strange.

This other me, this intensely real me, floated gently upwards like a feather towards a glowing brightness that was without shape or any physical dimension. As I floated I gazed down placidly on the scene below. I could see myself – my physical body – lying on a trolley, and I could see the doctors and nurses working frantically on a corpse – my body.

One was busy setting up another IV, someone else was monitoring my ECG, another was inserting a proper urinary catheter while at 'my' head someone had inserted an endotracheal tube and was hitching it up to a ventilator.

I looked down on them in complete detachment, tranquility, almost with wry amusement. I was strangely apart from everything I knew and loved, including family and work. I felt at ease.

At this point someone pushed his way towards my body from the side. He looked like a circus clown. His face was streaked with white paint, his eyes bulged and his dark mop of hair was spiked in a fashion that only became popular decades later. A voice thundered from somewhere. These are the exact words I heard. 'Go away, he is not yours'.

Above me the brightness began to fade to a soft glow until it disappeared completely and I reluctantly drifted down to the body below.

The monitor began to stabilise and the defib machine was switched off. I was in sinus rhythm, my blood pressure started to climb back to normal and my blood oxygenation flickered around 90 per cent. I would sleep deeply for some time.

This was my out-of-world experience, no different to that told by hundreds of others. You can say it was due to hypoxia of the brain or you can say it was my soul or spirit leaving my body. But whatever you say, you can know it did happen to me and is neither exaggerated nor doctored in any way.

The next three weeks were spent in isolation. I was not aware of anything much for the first 7–ten days, but when I emerged from my torpor the first person I saw was Doreen, my dear wife, sitting patiently beside me. She had flown over from Dublin and was my constant bedside companion for the remainder of my stay. My diagnosis had been confirmed. I had been infected with louse borne typhus.

Louse borne typhus is truly a disease of dirt, of overcrowding, of unsanitary conditions. It claimed more lives in the great Irish famine of the 1840s than did starvation and has been more lethal than bullets in wars from the 1400s on. The doctors told me it was the first case of typhus recorded in Switzerland in the twentieth century – so at least I had made a bit of history for them. I could have nipped it in the bud had I used almost any other antibiotic except Septrin.

I was extremely lucky to survive and, as I write this more than 30 years later, I know I owe those years to the love and dedication of everyone who took care of me in 1985.

It was a very hard time for my family even after I was flown home. I spent the first few weeks in Our Lady of Lourdes Hospital in Drogheda recuperating, but it took several months before I recovered fully. Recover I did; yet I was not ready to go on another adventure for several more years.

Afterwards I wondered how and when I was bitten by typhus infected lice, while no one else in our team got infected.

I have come to the conclusion that I got infected by lice from the dying children that I held closely in my arms while I infused fluid into the jugular vein. I took these children straight in as emergency cases from the queues outside. There was no time to wash or disinfest them, and they still wore the same filthy louse-ridden clothes that they had used for months.

Famine Post-Script: Menigstu Goes

The corrupt rule of Haile Selassie was followed by the corrupt rule of Haile Mariam Mengistu. Both started with high ideals and both descended into despotic tyranny. Today Ethiopia and Eritrea – which regained its independence after Mengistu fled in 1991 – stand as two proud and independent nations despite ongoing poverty and difficult climate challenges.

It was some consolation for the people of these countries when, in 2006, Mengistu was convicted of genocide *in abstentia* by an Ethiopian court. This conviction related primarily the *Red Terror* years in which Mengistu had the dead bodies of those whom he mistrusted thrown on the streets. However, the conviction was in some ways a meaningless gesture in that Robert Mugabe immediately granted Mengistu and many *Derg* families asylum in Zimbabwe. Indeed, he treated the deposed dictator as an honoured guest and refused point blank to extradite him.

As for me, I eventually convalesced at home before resuming work in the University in Galway. I had made it. And I am now immune to typhus!

However to this day I regret that my time was so short in Ethiopia and that I contributed so little to relieving the suffering of the people there.

CHAPTER 11
EGYPTIAN INTERLUDE 1992

Most Europeans and North Americans fly south to Egypt across the Mediterranean. My youngest daughter Danielle and I were exceptions in that we flew north from Kampala to Cairo, up the African continent so to speak, rather than down from Europe.

I had just completed a working stint in Kampala during which I wrote a report on the current status of HIV/AIDS status in Uganda for the WHO. This gave me an opportunity to take one of my children with me and Danielle was the chosen one. She was barely 21 years old and ready for life. Our detour home via Cairo was to be a special treat. But unfortunately our budget was very depleted after our stay in Uganda since we had given away almost all we had. And this was in spite of staying free of charge with the Franciscan sisters in Nsambya Hospital.

Nonetheless, we were in great form as we boarded the plane in Entebbe and would have been in better form had I searched the front pocket of my suitcase where Sr Anne Needham had slipped a 100-dollar note, probably guessing our financial plight. We only found this gift after returning to Ireland, but oh, how we could have used it in Egypt. By coincidence Anne was a sister of Michael Needam a friend of mine living in Galway.

We arrived in Cairo airport in a good mood, excited at the prospect of seeing the pyramids, the Sphinx and the Valley of the Kings. Our first task was to visit the airport tourist office where they recommended us to take the shuttle bus into the city, which would stop near Ramses Square, the ideal place to find a good inexpensive hotel.

As a result, we disappointed hordes of taxi drivers who crowded around us and who assumed we would take a taxi to the city. Instead we made for a shabby looking bus that had 'Shuttle to Cairo' painted on its side.

Our good mood was tested from the moment we stepped on board. For starters the driver fumbled with our money and I was not sure what I was paying him except that I was probably paying too much. Then we found we had to stand. There was no empty seat available and enormous women covered in black from head to toe occupied the few seats that were there. This did not worry us unduly. It is hard to sit comfortably at eye level with other peoples' backsides. Especially when it is hot, everyone is sweating profusely and the majority of them are blowing *flatus vulgaris* right at you. So we stood, squeezed against one another, all jostling together, in one swaying sticky organic mass. There was much loud talking between the passengers and between the passengers and the driver who was clearly irritated by one burly Egyptian who seemed to be asking him to detour so that he could get off at his home. The driver won the argument and the burly man descended into a scowley silence.

Luckily the journey only took around 30 minutes before we lurched to a halt. Those who stood now had the advantage and got off first. It was like disentangling a ball of wool. We were all sticky and sweaty as we peeled off and landed on the hot sidewalk. Danielle and I pushed our way out oblivious to people we elbowed in the process. We had little luggage yet, as if by magic, many children appeared promising to carry our things and show us a 'good cheap hotel'.

The sights and sounds of Cairo are unique and cannot be adequately described. It is like being dropped into a tin can with someone beating on the lid. Radios blare from shops; cars, buses, lorries and motorbikes rev and backfire and blow their horns continuously. In the midst of this drivers lean out windows and shout imprecations at one another. Ambulances and police cars chase along with their sirens on and you begin to wonder how anyone gets anywhere without being knocked down.

For there are crowds of people of all sizes, shapes and ages thronging the sidewalks and darting with incredible heroism across roads which are packed with every kind of motorised and non-motorised conveyance imaginable.

Cairo is alive.

A lodging for the next few nights was our first aim, and since we found that we had been left off around the corner from Ramses Square, our search began immediately.

The most striking thing about Ramses Square was the giant 11-metre high, 83-ton statute of Ramses 11, which dominated the centre. Colonel Nasser – the same colonel who had successfully defied Britain and France over the ownership of the Suez Canal in 1956 – had it transported there a year earlier. Nassar literally screwed the six pieces of the original statue together so that it could stand erect once more, and installed it on a three metre high plinth with a lovely fountain in front where people could congregate, talk, lounge and simply pass the time in the shadow of the great man.

Ramses 11

Ramses 11 (Ozymandial in Greek writings) was the greatest of all the Pharaohs. He lived the longest and built the most temples and cities and waged the most successful wars. But had he done none of these things, I think he would have been famous because of the beautiful Nefertari, the favourite of his eight wives. It was on our agenda to see the burial tombs of Ramses 11 and Nefertari in the Valleys of the Kings and Queens when we visited Luxor. Of course, both tombs had been looted long ago.

It was with Nefertari that Ramses travelled to Abu Simbel in Nubia to open a great rock temple – to himself. The Swiss traveller Johan Buckhardt could hardly contain his excitement when he discovered it buried in sand in 1813. This was the same Buckhardt who discovered Petra, the 'red city' of the Nabataens, the previous year. Those were exciting times indeed.

Danielle and I were lucky enough to see the original 3,300-year-old granite statue of Ramses 11 in Ramses Square. Young as Danielle was, she gazed in wonder at the massive statue, and we both felt overawed by its sheer size, age and exquisite workmanship. It has since been transported to Giza and from there to the new Grand Egyptian Museum in order to prevent further damage from the weather, urban pollution and vibration from the metro below and the traffic at street level.

We walked around the square becoming more and more dismayed as we saw one grubby hotel after another. But we were tired, hot, thirsty and travel weary, and in need of some-place to rest. So we settled on what seemed a decent enough place. If we got a front room high enough we would be looking directly at Ramses side face and across to the other side of the square.

The hotel we chose seemed clean and respectable if a little run down. It fulfilled three important requirements for tired impecunious travellers; it was cheap, the room appeared clean and there was a bolt on the inside of the door. The room we were allotted was on the very top floor, 23 stories up. In those days we never thought of what would happen in case of a fire.

The elevator looked a bit dodgy and on the advice of a lethargic but helpful Egyptian who was sitting behind a small desk in the little foyer, we climbed the stairs. 'Its quicker and safer' he reassured us. I cannot call him a receptionist, nor can I call the place he sat in a real foyer, but he looked kind, had a big round smiling face and I wonder in retrospect if he really believed that we were father and daughter staying together in the same room for he gave me a knowing wink which was somewhat disconcerting.

That first night we were so tired we did not care what anyone thought, yet we were alert enough to notice the many small dark stains on our bed sheets. I knew immediately that we had the company of bed bugs, but our defences were down and we were just glad to be somewhere with a secure lock on the door. Our room – technically a penthouse – was really a garret, with a sloping ceiling obviously following the slope of the roof. A small dormer window was inserted in the roof through which we could hear but not see the people and traffic on the square below. The bonus was that we had a privileged view of the top of Ramses' head – if we stood on tip toes and squinted through the less dirty parts of the window pane.

The Railway Station stood on the far side of the square, directly across from our hotel. This was – and remains – the major transport hub in Cairo. It connects buses and trains not only with the rest of Egypt but also with the local metro system, and so, in a very practical way, Ramses Square is an excellent base for the tourist.

Unfortunately the hustle and bustle of the square, where the commerce of day continues through the night, does not make for a restful sleep. And if you think that taking a stroll round the Square will help, then you are wrong. Any foreigner, and especially anyone who looks like a tourist, stands out incongruously and conspicuously among the white robed locals.

This can be intimidating but the railway station is even more intimidating. You are continually pestered there by people seeking to sell you something, offering you a great rate of exchange, or promising to act as your personal guide to Cairo. Many offer to bring you to places where you can indulge any desire you wish. This is all very understandable when you consider how poor people are and how every foreigner is seen as a multimillionaire ready to be relieved of his or her money. Despite all this we slept well.

Next morning we travelled on the metro to the centre of the city. It was the first time we had ever seen women-only carriages and, despite what Google says, the Cairo metro had them as far back as 1992. The metro took us – in a mixed carriage – almost directly to the Cairo museum, the real object of our first days outing. Here we viewed many of the ancient artefacts of Egypt but the whole subject of Egyptology is so complex and was so new to us that we soon got totally confused by all the gods and goddesses.

Naturally everyone was crowding around Tutankhamen and we joined in with a Canadian tour so that we had the pleasure of an excellent guide at no cost. Later we made a deal with a taxi driver to bring us to Giza next day. The taxi man's name was Alexander. Strange how you remember odd inconsequential details from the past and forget many important things. Well, anyway, Alexander was a big guy, had a Mercedes taxi – of which he was clearly proud – and gave us the history of his own family – in which we were not interested – rather than a history of Egypt, which was what we wanted. However he did bring us safely to the Pyramids and to the Sphinx and, although we parked a long way from them we enjoyed the experience thoroughly.

We thought the Sphinx was the most impressive of the monuments there. There is something eternal and timeless in the way the Sphinx looks out across the desert. It seems to mock the arrogance of modern man and serves as a reminder of how insignificant and transient we are. It also makes one wonder if our present civilisation will pass away and crumble like the great civilisations of old.

What a shame that most of the population of the world never get to see other countries and experience other cultures. I suppose I have been luckier than most in this regard although I did not appreciate my good fortune at the time.

Luxor

Two nights later we left our bed-bug hotel, crossed the road, and took the overnight bus to Luxor. In ancient times Luxor was known as Thebes, a city that had been the capital of an immensely rich empire for almost a thousand years. Homer refers to Thebes in the Iliad as 'the city of a hundred gates.... which only the grains of the desert surpass the abundance of wealth contained therein.' It housed half a million people, an incredible number at the time, and all worshipped Amon who was expected to protect it from the predators that stalked its every side.

Ezekiel prophesied its downfall – as he had done for Memphis – and what a fall it had. Its destruction was complete and terrible as wave after wave of barbarians butchered its people and pillaged its treasures.

Yet enough of ancient Thebes remains to lure travellers from every corner of the earth and both Danielle and myself were as keen as any Egyptologist to see this city of cities for ourselves.

However our choice of travelling there by overnight bus was a mistake. The bus was noisy, crowded and bumpy. Most of all it was cold. Nighttime in the desert can be very cold, and you feel this more acutely because of the great contrast to the heat of the day. In addition, because we sat near the front door, we were exposed not only to a constant blast of cold air but also to intermittent clouds of dust and sand, whipped up by a desert wind.

The driver kept swigging something from a bottle stuck down beside his seat and had the radio turned on to loud music, which was neither Western nor Eastern in character, but the lowest denominator of both, an amalgam of the worst of both kinds. Nonetheless the other passengers did not object, indeed they seemed to like it. Then, after an hour or so, they covered their heads in woollen blankets, contorted their bodies to fit the shape of the seats and removed their shoes, before promptly snoring the night away.

We drove on steadily through the endless desert and an endless sleepless night until the first grey streaks of dawn appeared on the eastern horizon and the stars went out one by one.

It was worth it in the end. We got our second wind so to speak as we entered Luxor and got an early morning glimpse of the Nile. This was the same Nile I had seen in Jinga and in Khartoum, the mother river that has sustained so many millions of people and so many empires and dynasties in the past. We both stared at its broad waters in fascination as our bus finally rumbled to a stop.

While in Cairo we had arranged to stay in a little hotel in the centre of Luxor. The guy in reception in our Cairo lodging had recommended it. 'My cousin owns the place and will take good care of you.' Once more it was another dingy affair but this time there were no bed bugs. It was but a short walk from the Nile and not far from the Old Winter Palace hotel, made famous as the place where Agatha Christie wrote *Death on the Nile* between the two world wars. It was also but a stone's throw from the Luxor Temple which, on its own account, would have been a star attraction, but for the nearby Temple at Karnak.

You get a glimpse of the magnificence of Karnak in the film version of Agatha Christie's book, where someone pushes a massive boulder over the top of a tall column in order to kill someone else below. Happily no such incident occurred when we were there; however, much as the official guides might have wanted to do away with us. For we joined with other strays like ourselves who hovered on the edges of different groups, listening to their prattle unashamedly. No book, no pictures, no telling can approach the experience of actually seeing and touching these ancient monuments. Nor is there any way to convey the depth and intensity of the emotions evoked by walking between row after row of mathematically precise towering columns of solid stone just as the Egyptians did three and a half thousand years ago. We still gawk in wonder at the massive columns, arches and statues. The atmosphere permeates every one of your senses and you seem – not just to share – but also to become one with the spirits of those who have passed this way and gazed on exactly the same things down the millennia.

We returned to our hotel that evening but not before we sat on the terrace of the Old Winter Palace and ate delicious tilapia washed down by cold local beer, all the time watching the sun gracefully dip beneath the horizon. As day faded so did the figures plying feluccas, skiffs and dhows on the river become silhouettes and then drift into darkness.

Soon it was night. The dark heavens glittered and glimmered with a quilt of twinkling stars and the pale moon rose serenely, almost lazily, to suffuse everything in a silver glow.

One can understand the ancients believing that the Nile was not only the mother of all rivers but also the mother of mankind.

Next day we were up bright and early. We walked to the river and rented bicycles and waited to take the ferry to the opposite side, where we planned to visit the Valley of the Kings and the Valley of the Queens.

I think the fare across was in the region of five cents, so for once we were getting something well within our means. The ferry trip was uneventful but you never know about ferries. There seems to be a report of a foreign ferry sinking somewhere every week. Arthur Moore, the chief anaesthetist in Merlin Park Hospital when I was working there, once asked the question 'What is the most trivial and uninteresting headline you can find in a newspaper?'

Many of us had heard him ask this question before but he would shock those who had not, by replying to his own question 'Overcrowded ferry sinks in Bangladesh, only 49 drowned'. And sadly Arthur was probably right.

Well our ferry was overcrowded but fortunately did not sink.

Yet we were glad to disembark, as there was little comfort in being squashed together on the deck of an ancient groaning boat, which had obviously been discarded as obsolete years before by some other Company.

Once safely on *terra firma* we mounted our bikes and headed towards the famous Valleys full of hope and expectation. The day was getting warmer but not yet hot, so we were able to cycle along freely with golden desert on both sides and a smooth blacktop beneath or wheels.

The first major artifacts we encountered were the Colossi of Memnon. These are two massive statues made of red sandstone that were erected by the Pharaoh Amenhotep 111rd in the fourteenth century BC. They are all that remains of the largest temple ever built in Egypt, even larger than those at Karnak or Abu Simbel. The figures themselves are badly eroded above the waist but you can see they gaze steadily in the direction of the Nile, as if worshipping the river that brings fertility to the soil and wealth to the people of Egypt. The major figure is of the man-god Amenhotep himself. The lesser ones depict his mother and wife and the god of the Nile.

Once past the Colossi we made our way to the Valleys, parked and locked our bikes, and followed the signs to any tombs that were open that day.

There was an Egyptian guide in each tomb who prattled off names and statistics and who waited with his hand out for a tip at each exit. We ended up totally confused but duly impressed by the inventiveness of the tomb builders and the cleverness of the wall drawings and the sheer effrontery of the guides.

We were all the time uneasy about the safety of our bikes so, after visiting a few tombs, we decided to go back to Luxor. Dare I say the unsayable: once the average you and I have seen one tomb we have seen them all!

It was now well into the afternoon and we had no desire to miss the 6 p.m. ferry. The cycle back was not easy. It was a scorching hot ride without shade or shelter, but we made it back to the Nile, happy, tired and hot, and looking forward to a good long sleep as soon as we hit the bed.

Early next morning we walked to Luxor Railway Station and caught the train to Cairo. This time we went first class and had nice lounge seats with clear views of the rolling countryside as we sped towards the capital. We now felt like well-seasoned travellers and knew exactly where we were going once we reached Cairo. The train ran smoothly, coke was available from the steward and altogether we were a content pair.

The concierge in our hotel in Ramses Square greeted us like old friends and listened enrapt to the story of our trip to Luxor. 'I will jolly well go there sometime myself' he chuckled. Or words to that effect.

The man had never been outside Cairo, he had never seen his cousin's hotel. I wondered if he had ever been outside Ramses Square.

We slept well that night – ignoring bed bug stains – and next day flew back to Ireland.

CHAPTER 12
SOUTH SUDAN 1993

South Sudan is as different from North Sudan as can be imagined. The North is dry, hot, arid and mostly desert. The sand hills of the Sahara roll on endlessly. You feel near the beginning of things as you stand among these fingers of time that, although they seem everlasting, change continuously in shape and form, height and colour at the caprice of the hot wind and the passage of the sun across the blue North African sky.

The north is a land of flowing white robes, caravan trains and stately camels, and of dust and sand. Minarets dot the skyline of its cities and towns, and the call to prayer six times a day is to be heard wherever you go, even in the smallest hamlet.

The people are fine boned, good looking and pale skinned. On the streets of Khartoum, they may be noisy and even aggressive to one another but they will always help foreigners and go out of their way to protect you if you are respectful of their culture. In the desert, they are gentle, welcoming and courteous.

The South is completely different. Here Islam has made hardly any impact. The prevailing culture is based on animism and the majority of people are, at least nominally, Christian. Tribally – where I worked in the Kongor province – most people are Dinkas but several smaller tribes exist notably the Nuer and the Murle.

For me the word 'very' pre-fixes the attributes of the Dinkas, for they are very tall, very colourful, very elegant, very graceful and very spiritual. While normally a quiet people, when aroused they can be very angry, passionate and even very frightening.

The southern Sudanese are dark skinned and seem to have little in common, either racially or in their disposition, with the inhabitants of Khartoum.

A Little History

The Egyptian conquest of present day South Sudan began in earnest in the 1820s. It was a patchy conquest and most people in the south followed their own tribal chiefs and were hardly aware of Cairo. But the Khedives eyed this vast land with an acquisitive eye and soon allied themselves to Britain for whom the golden era of empire was approaching its zenith. As a result, an Anglo-Egyptian authority was set up to rule all Sudan, north and south, and this was propped up by British guns.

With the British came the traders and Christian missionaries. The latter made little progress in the Muslim north but established themselves firmly in the less developed south. Indeed neither the Egyptian or British rulers paid much attention to the south because of its geographical isolation and its disease-ridden climate.

In practise, real power over Sudan as a whole lay in the hands of the Mahdists. The Mahdists' aim was to create a pure Islamic state in which the 'Mahdi', their supreme chief, would free the people from the bonds of the degenerate Egyptians and the misguided British.

And the Mahdists would have succeeded but for the money and modern weaponry of their opponents. Tales of Kitchener and 'the Mahdi' regaled the British public in Victorian times but all this faded away in the twentieth century until finally, in 1956, the Republic of Sudan was created as in independent State into which an almost overlooked South Sudan became fully 'integrated' – on paper.

One can safely say that there was never a time when South Sudan enjoyed peace either before or after 1956. If it was not wars against neighbouring countries then it was intertribal wars, and the latter have continued long after South Sudan itself became a fully sovereign country, following a referendum among its people in 2011. Africa's newest country had been born.

The details of atrocities, tortures, pillage, village burning and every crime you can think of have been reported to an incredulous but apathetic outside world and, as usual, the toothless UN simply passed pious resolutions condemning this behaviour as 'unacceptable' or labelling it as an effort at 'genocide' while human rights groups thumped their chests in futile outrage.

South Sudan remains riven with disease, disaster and division to this day.

A Little Geography

South Sudan is totally landlocked and is cut off from the rest of Sudan by an immense swamp of almost 1,600 km², called the Sudd. The Sudd, or more properly the *Al-Sudd*, is formed by the White Nile as it wends its way north, and is an impenetrable labyrinth of overgrown waterways and morasses which form a natural barrier that makes navigation of the river impossible.

The country is otherwise covered in rich tropical rainforest and lush grasses and has a huge variety of wildlife, probably more varied than anywhere else in Africa. Beneath the soil lie rich mineral deposits and that most precious commodity, oil, black gold.

Yet despite all its potential, South Sudan is among the least developed countries in the world. Its very inaccessibility and the high prevalence of tropical diseases have deterred development. Indeed South Sudan is regarded by some as an anachronism rather than as a modern nation with a potential for growth, prosperity and power.

I Go with John O'Shea's GOAL

When I went to the South Sudan in the early 2000s, I knew nothing of the politics or history of this troubled place. I had volunteered to do a three months' stint there as I had heard that people were starving, disease was rife and a civil war was raging.

I went with GOAL, a humanitarian group set up by my old friend John O'Shea. John was both liked and disliked.

He was liked because he had dedicated his life to helping the oppressed in the Third World. And he was admired because he went out personally to poor and often dangerous places, set up his organisation on the spot and employed as many locals as possible. He had boundless energy, tremendous drive and had the 'get it done at all costs' philosophy that one associates with Munster Rugby. He was the Ryanair of humanitarians. He took little money for himself yet got the job done speedily and efficiently.

John was always a keen sportsman and had been a sports journalist with the Irish Press group for many years. So it was no coincidence that he focused his fundraising around sports events. This turned out to be an inspired move as sportsmen and women everywhere flocked to support him. Consequently, he had many ardent supporters who helped him raise funds both in Ireland and abroad, often by tapping into sporting events and sponsoring sporting activities such as the famous Goal Mile race.

However, on the debit side, he was somewhat feared by those who found him difficult to work with. His autocratic style and always-being-right mentality upset them. He seemed to take little account of personal feelings and did not suffer fools gladly. Personal diplomacy was not his strong point.

Thus, many criticised him – behind his back – because of the dictatorial way in which he ran his organisation. Of course, this was the way to get things done quickly and efficiently and John knew that and made no apology for it.

John was never short of courage. His open criticism of Governments both here and overseas did not endear him to the establishment and his forthright accusations of the misuse of Irish Aid to Uganda was a thorn in the side of diplomatic relationships between Ireland and that country.

Furthermore, he made people, ordinary people, feel uncomfortable by the accusatory and uncompromising way he spoke and wrote. He made them feel guilty for living comfortable lives when so many people were being crushed by hunger, famine and war. One of Donald Trump's slogans seems to describe John's attitude, and I paraphrase: *You cannot be honest without offending people.*

I first met John in Thailand in 1979. He had just filled a Boeing 707 with food and medical supplies and delivered it there for distribution among refugees from Kampuchea. John had founded GOAL two years earlier when he raised money for the poor of Kolkata (Calcutta), but his public image only really took off after his involvement in Cambodia.

His visits to the 'field' were whirlwinds that left his volunteers, which we called *Goalies*, exhausted. Even physically, he

was a ball of fire. I remember one evening, oh it was somewhere in Africa, I cannot remember where, when he suggested,
no... he *decided*... that we all play basketball. We duly obeyed,
tired though we were, after a long day's work. He raced around
knocking people down as if he were a schoolboy and I know I
only lasted the pace for ten minutes after being pushed by our
boss to the ground several times.

Whatever his faults, this fanatic sportsman, this fanatic
do-gooder and this larger-than-life man contributed more to
relieving suffering than any other person I ever met. And, on a
personal level, you would have to like him.

I know that I liked and respected him despite his alleged
dislike of doctors. He argued rightly that nurses are more
hands-on, more knowledgeable and generally more useful
than doctors in delivering emergency relief – a view with
which I concur.

Daily Run from 'Loki' to Kongor

Unfortunately, the security position in South Sudan was so bad
that we could not base ourselves there but had to fly in daily
from Lokichokio – which we all called 'Loki' – a small town
in Turkana in northern Kenya. The UN had a large base there
and GOAL was just one of the several agencies it housed. The
majority served the huge refugee camp in Kakuma, with just a
few taking the risk of entering South Sudan. Concern Ireland
along with GOAL were among these, but even Concern pulled
out at one point – wisely in my view – whereas GOAL just kept
going in.

Chuck was our pilot. Chuck was a tanned strong young
man who called himself a 'white Rhodesian' (Zimbabwean).
His family had lived in Africa for several generations and he
would not let go of the old ways. To me he was straight from

'Out of Africa' and depicted a breed of arrogant white person who was an anachronism even in those days. But on a one-to-one basis, Chuck was helpful and concerned and extremely respectful for people irrespective of their background. Chuck said he was doing this work for the money and did not pretend otherwise.

Chuck was a good pilot. Our landing on a grass strip in Kongor was always bumpy and dangerous, but Chuck managed it beautifully every time

Once the plane stopped, one of us would open the door and jump down on the ground. Willing hands stretched out to help us as we landed and a group of locals scrambled to carry whatever bags of rice and maize and powdered milk we had with us. Then the lot of us would walk to the 'town' about 200 metres away.

All the while local children scampered beside us, giggling and smiling and chatting noisily among themselves. We tried to bring some little treat for them. A small piece of chocolate was a prize worth waiting for, and even the adults held out their hands in a shameless competition with the young ones as four or five Goalie nurses plus myself tramped along.

Chuck always stayed in the plane with instructions to sound a loud klaxon at the first sign of danger. On hearing this, we were to drop everything and run back to the plane, which was ready to take off at a moment's notice.

In time, we all got to like Chuck and occasionally he would let one of the nurses or myself take over the controls – for a few minutes – which was a great bonus and very exciting. And never once did any of us lose our cool.

However, I did once lose my cool in another sense while waiting to board Chuck's plane early one morning. Two nurses and I were standing close to the plane waiting to get aboard as it was being re-fuelled. A long-faced dour Scotsman was filling the plane with high-octane jet gasoline and at the same time had a lighted cigarette in his mouth. You could see the waving mist of petrol in the early morning sun and I was certain that the gas would take light and that we would all be burned alive.

I turned to Chuck and said 'Chuck … this nutter … he'll blow up the whole place up if he does not put out that cigarette.' Chuck just shrugged his shoulders but then unexpectedly turned to the guy and told him to 'put out that bloody cigarette' with an unmistakable edge on his voice. There was a moment of eye-to-eye confrontation but Chuck won the day. I walked away happy that I had been vindicated but conscious too that I was getting snake eyes from the Scotsman. The nurses said nothing but I think they were happy that their doctor had showed some guts.

Our daily flight lasted perhaps 30–40 minutes and took us over the Jonglei canal. I should explain that this canal had been first mooted by Sir William Garstin in 1907 but only started in 1978 and was not yet complete. The purpose was to divert waters from the vast Sudd to irrigate northern Sudan and southern Egypt. The scale of the work would be colossal and the benefits enormous to everyone – except those living in South Sudan. So it came as no surprise when the Sudanese Peoples Liberation Army (SPLA) wrecked the project before the last 120 km was excavated.

We passed over this strange snake-like gash in the earth each day, with little thought of those who had laboured on it for so long. We could even see one of the rusting giant German excavators, which sooner or later the earth would entomb in a snub to the arrogance of man.

At that time, the SPLA was in charge and so we were in rebel territory and in fear of attack by the regular Sudanese army at any time. Chuck was well aware of this and stuck close by his plane ready for a quick exit at the first sign of danger.

Kongor

I need not describe the town of Kongor itself. It was an awful place. It was pretty terrible when it was built but was a thousand times worse after its recent 'liberation' by the SPLA. Houses were mostly roofless, walls were puckered with bullet and mortar holes, the people had a furtive, hunted and fearful look, and in general, only the children seemed to have any life in them.

Even the prisoners – there was a kind of prison there – were lifeless. They sat about, outside the prison, almost naked and obviously half-starved, making no attempt to escape. 'Where would I go?' one prisoner asked me.

It was true. The SPLA had mined all the roads leading out of the town, and besides, the same prisoner told me he came from Port Sudan, a thousand miles to the north.

Much of my time in Kongor was taken up treating minor tropical illnesses and dishing out ORS for diarrhoea to both adults and children. I had a fair amount of antibiotics and I used what I had liberally. Deworming, delousing and giving iron and vitamin preparations; checking ante-natals, assessing nutritional status, doing wt./ht. charts and doling out food in a way that everyone was registered so that cheating was minimal; the nurses and I shared all these tasks. Together, we scrubbed the floors and whitewashed the walls of our Clinic so that after a few weeks the place began to look respectable. So much for the glamour of working in the midst of famine and war.

Guinea Worm

It was the first time I had seen so many cases of 'guinea worm'. The condition is caused by drinking water contaminated with a flea that contains the larvae of the parasite. Once inside our bodies the larvae mature over 8–10 months until mating occurs after which the now useless males perish. Finally, the mature gravid females penetrate the skin and discharge their eggs into freshwater.

Often several worms come out at the same time and it is a most distressing thing to see them wagging and writhing as if looking around to see where they are. Once the worm begins to emerge, infection can set in and so the disease may present as single or multiple abscesses, with the body of the guinea worm stuck deep down in the midst of the pus. The cycle of infection and re-infection is perpetuated in the women and children who go to the well to fetch water.

Even today there is no specific treatment. All one can do is try to extract the intact worm. This is done – and has been done for generations – by winding the worm around a small stick as it emerges, and carefully turning the stick a little each day so that the entire worm can be eventually pulled out.

But if there was a clean water supply, so that no one need fetch water from a contaminated well, we would have the final answer to this totally avoidable condition.

Col John Garang

On one of our visits to Kongor Col John Garang, the founder of the SPLA, made a fleeting appearance. He was on his way to Juba, the present capital of South Sudan.

Much has been written about Garang and his wife Rebecca, some of it good and some of it bad. In my view – based on nothing more than listening to Africans talking – both will be remembered as heroes who devoted their lives to the betterment of the ordinary people of South Sudan.

Garang died in a helicopter crash in 2005. Some dispute the circumstances of this crash, which has led to much argument at the time.

Kola Boof

The speaker/author Kola Boof has been one of the most notable supporters of the Garangs. She is best known as the self-confessed ex-mistress of Osama Bin Laden. However, she also knew Garang when she was a child and later became an active supporter of the SPLA. An American couple had adopted her after her parents were murdered following their reports of witnessing slavery in the Sudan. Boof actually cites her father telling Garang that there were 'Arabs selling Dinka and Nuer children like cattle' (interview 2005).

Had Garang lived, he would have been sad to see the ongoing strife and misery of Africa's most recent nation. Yet he would have been proud to see that little Juba has grown from a tiny settlement in 1922 to a thriving city of nearly half a million people today and, doubtless prouder still of the country's economy, which has been lifted by vast revenues from local oil wells.

Rebecca, John's widow, went on to have a distinguished political career but fell foul of John's successor, Salva Kiir, who, in 2013, put her under house arrest. After a voluntary exile in Kenya for nearly two years, she returned amid jubilation to Juba in November 2015. She was 60 years old in 2016.

The Illegals?

In 1993, things were frankly awful in Kongor. And not much less awful for transient aid workers like us Goalies. Yet we kept

IMMANUEL HOSPITAL,

P. M. B. 10, EKET,

SOUTH EASTERN STATE OF NIGERIA.

Your Ref

Our Ref

15th February, 1969.

The Medical Officer i/c
St. Luke's Hospital,
Anua,
UYO.

In re. Mrs. Grace Joe.

I refer the above patient to you for what might be possible to do there. I do not wish to undertake such a big venture.

2. Mrs. Joe was fishing and got a living fish to slip into her throat by accident. This the second time I have known such an accident in my life time!

Medical Superintendent.

1. An unusual case

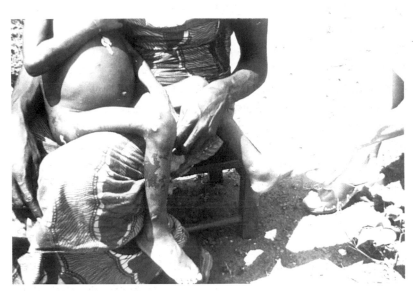

2. Kwashiorkor Biafra 1969

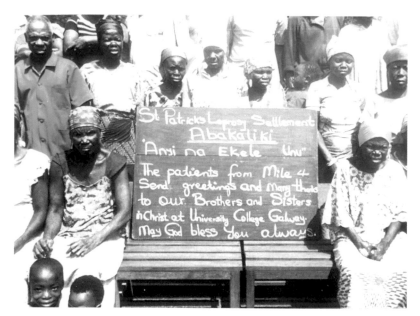

3. Lepers thank UCG students 1970

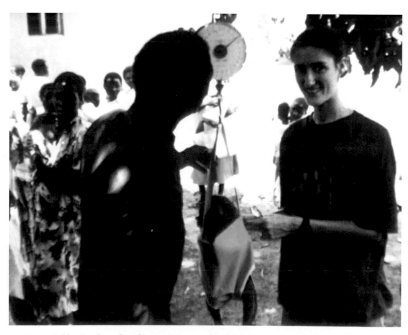

4. Danielle in bush clinic Uganda 1992

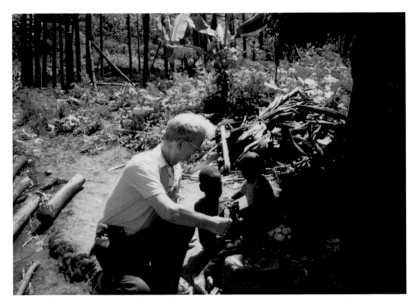

5. Rwanda 1994

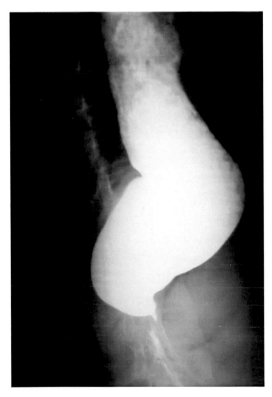

6. Dilated obstructed oesophagus, Chagas disease, Kampala 1983

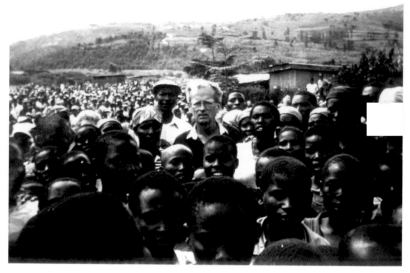

7. Anxious wait for food. Rwanda 1984

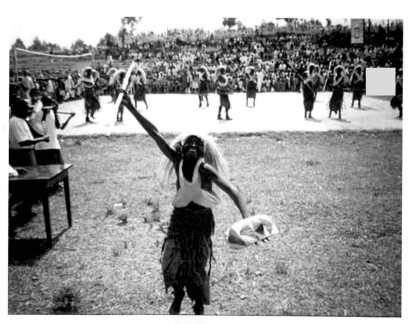

8. Thank you dance Rwanda 1985

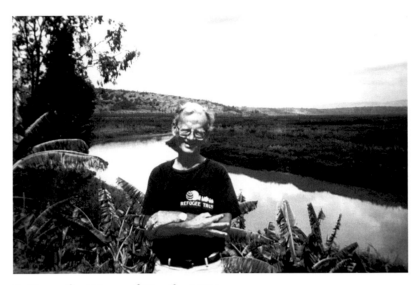

9. Rwanda. River of Death, 1994

10. Searching for gorillas, Rwanda

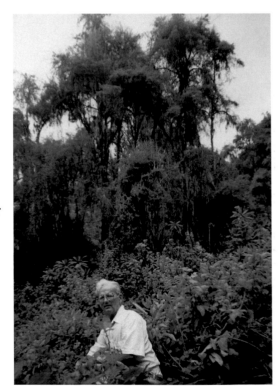

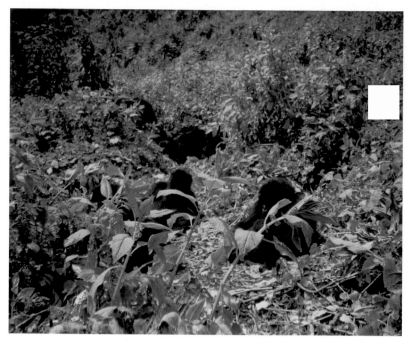

11. Gorillas in the mist, Rwanda

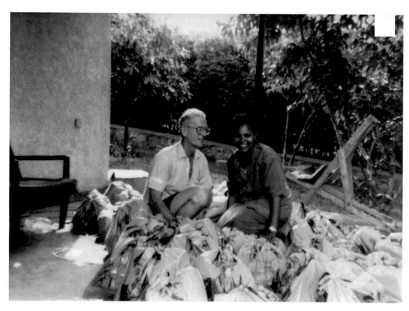

12. With Annette, Rwanda

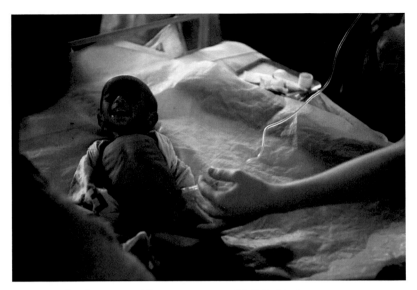

13. IP rehydration. Ethiopia 1984. Child died.

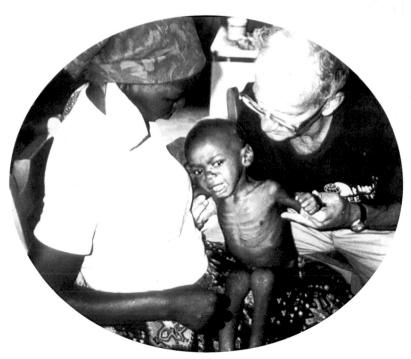

14. Pity not enough, Ethiopia 1984/5

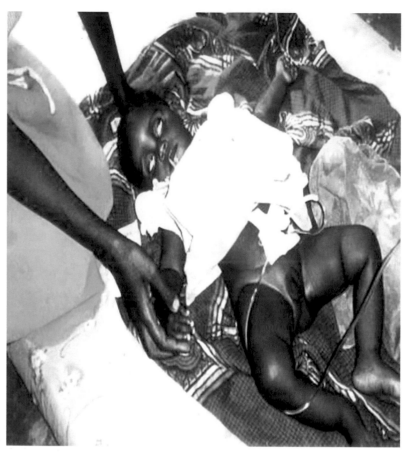

15. Ethiopian famine 1984/5. Child lived

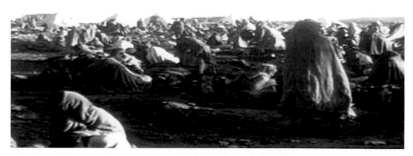

16. Sacking to keep out cold Ethiopia 1984/5

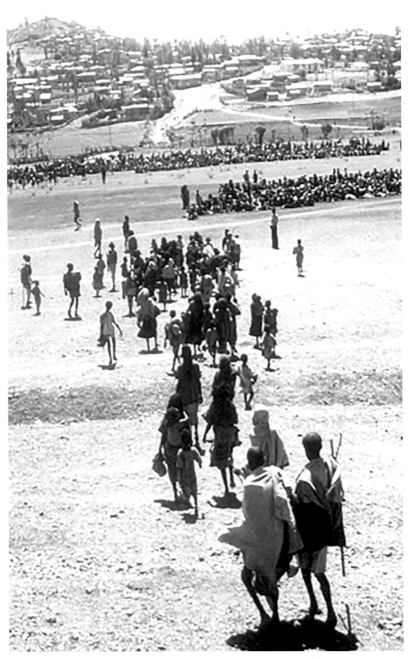

17. Biblical trek Ethiopia 1984/5

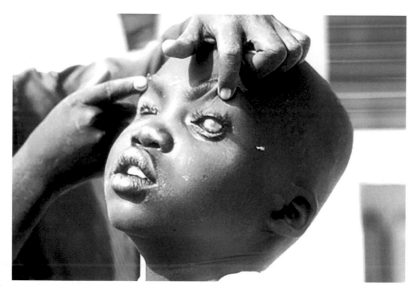

18. Trachoma

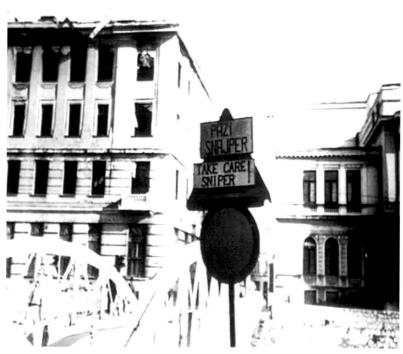

19. Daily commute Sarajevo 1995

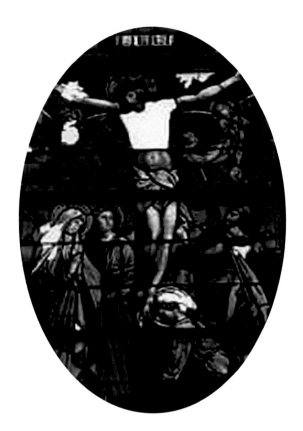

20. Shell blows out Christ's heart, Sarajevo

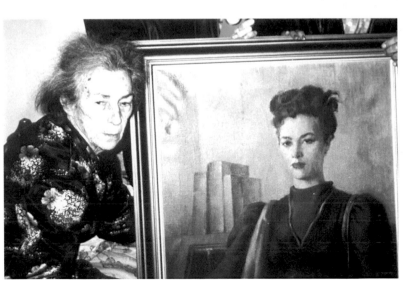

21. I was once a diva. Sarajevo 1995

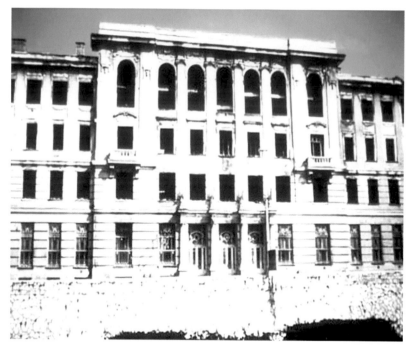

22. Post office, Sarajevo 1995

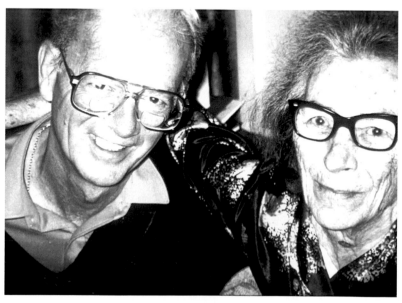

23. Home visit, Sarajevo

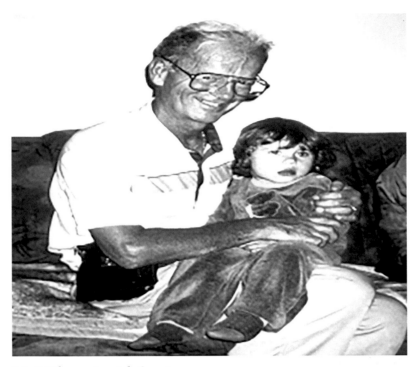

24. Little mute girl, Sarajevo

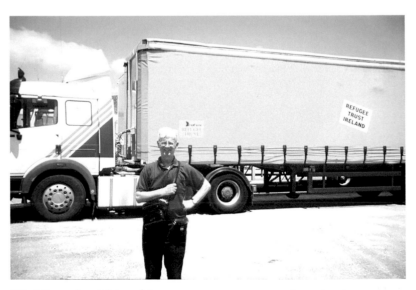

25. My only aid truck!

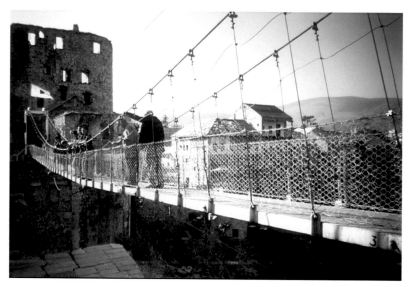

26. Temporary bridge, Mostar

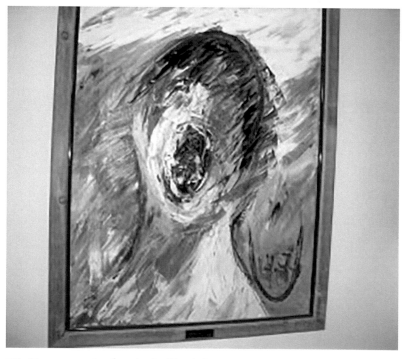

27. Kosovo cries by Anje Kapici

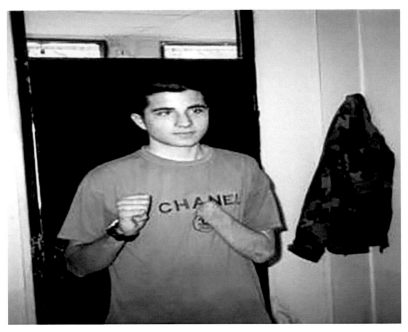

28. Why me? Kosovo 1999

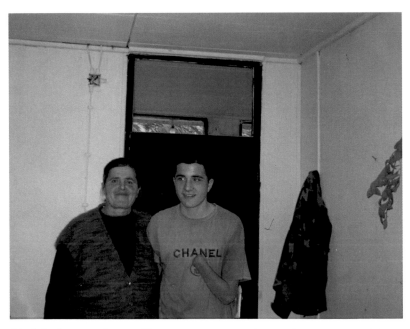

29. Mother and son, Kosovo

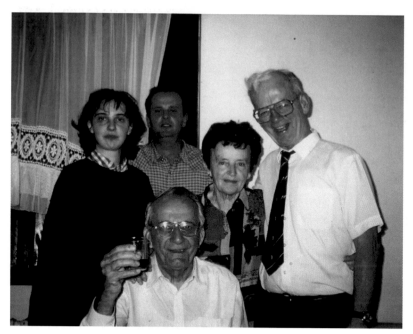

30. The 'Kočos'

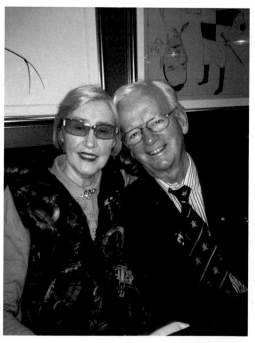

31. With Doreen in her last days

on going into this maelstrom of terror, intrigue and unpre-dictability on a daily basis oblivious to everything except our desire to be at least a presence for these forgotten people. That sounds very altruistic and noble but in reality we were just doing a job, a job that any doctor or nurse could do.

Yet I suspect few would have sneaked sick people across the border to Kenya – as we did – so they could be treated properly. Neither did I realise that I was involved in something dangerous until Chuck warned me. 'There may be no customs or security men at Loki airport… but be sure the word had got out about what you are doing. If I were you Dom I'd stop this immediately.'

At first I dismissed his warning because I believed I was doing the right thing and also because the remoteness of the area seemed to guarantee immunity from Kenyan law. But I later realised that I might be putting the whole humanitarian operation in jeopardy and that Chuck was being made an accomplice. That was a risk I could not take.

I stopped the practise. It was not an easy decision. These poor people were technically illegal immigrants and I was a people trafficker! Good law has no favourites – I suppose. Meantime we struggled on.

No Anaesthetic

We have all seen movies where legs are amputated, bullets removed or arrows pulled out from people without any anaesthetic.

I never thought I would have to do the same in real life. However, life can occasionally force us into doing things that go against every principle we hold dear and all of us must drink bitter wine from time to time.

My story concerns an operation on a prisoner in Kongor for whom there was no hope of escape. He had shown me his swollen right hand and immediately I detected the ominous presence of crepitus. Crepitus is a kind of crackling sound or squelchy sensation you feel when you squeeze bubble paper. In medicine, it signifies the presence of gas in the subcutaneous tissues. This is due to *Clostridium welchii*, a gas-producing organism, which is rapidly fatal and resistant to all our antibiotics.

My prisoner patient had the dreaded gas gangrene and the only hope to save his life was for me to amputate above the infected site.

Chuck had informed us that for security reasons, this was probably the last run we would make for the foreseeable future. I looked at the poor fellow and could see that already the signs of toxaemia were appearing. He had a rapid pulse, a high swinging fever, a severe headache and a hot clammy skin and was beginning to get confused.

A group of three or four prisoners led him into a small room off the main Clinic. This was a kind of storeroom – supposed to be secure – with wooden cupboards lining the walls in which we kept tablets (paracetamol, chloroquine and mebendazole), baby food, ORS and dried milk. There was also a rectangular wooden table there, which we would pull out into the main Clinic on Clinic days, and from which we would dispense drugs and food and any other item that we might have on a particular day. At break time, it became a dining table on which we could lay down our mugs of coffee.

Now it would be used as an operating table.

I had made up my mind. I would amputate through his right wrist leaving myself about an inch of healthy skin to close the stump. In this way, I did not need a saw. I had several very good surgical scissors capable of slicing through the wrist ligaments. But I only had five millilitre of novocaine, a local anaesthetic. This was barely enough to anaesthetise the skin, never mind the deeper structures. I had only one length of sterile catgut for tying off blood vessels and nothing with which to sew up the skin.

It is truly amazing how answers to ones problems appear from nowhere. There happened to be a rather odd Englishman who lived in Kongor for the past ten years. He was now in his seventies; tanned, lean and totally in love with Africa. He came to the rescue with some fine nylon, which he normally used in his beloved fishing rod. He offered it to me and said it would be ideal for stitching up skin. 'I have used it on myself ... a few times ... when there was no doctor around.' I believed him. This would have to do me. So I was set.

They lay the patient down on the table. We had no IV, no sterile packs, no proper lights (apart from sunlight through the back window) and no semblance of organisation. I remembered reading how the surgeons of old could remove a kidney stone without anaesthetic in 30 seconds or was it less?

I laid out my tools on a gauze pack, made sure my 'assistants' held the man's arm in a tight grip and I told my terrified patient that everything would be fine. Just a bit of pain and then it would be all over. I do not know if he understood me but our eyes communicated in a way far more meaningful than words. I said 'Jesus help me' to myself and mapped out my planned incision on his skin with the blue marker we used on notices outside the Clinic.

I then injected novocaine under the marked line and, after waiting for a few moments, cut all around the wrist as quickly as I could. One of our Goalie nurses held back the flaps I had made and then I got to the serious work of cutting through ligaments, disarticulating the wrist bones and tying off bleeders. I did not look at my man and I do not think I was aware of his screams. For I was told afterwards that he screamed before losing consciousness. The whole thing took between five and six minutes.

I was totally drained at the finish but now I could look at my patients face. He was wide-awake, and silent. Slowly he started to sit up. Against all protocol, we hugged each other. I knew there were tears in my eyes, but I did not care. I had nothing to say to him or to give him. Except, as I lay him back on the table, I became aware of his dirty, ragged T-shirt. It had probably been white once but was now mottled with brown stains and stiff with sweat and rain.

I took off my nice green T-shirt with GOAL printed on the back and gave it to him. His face lit up with a broad grin and his eyes smiled at me in a way that pierced all the cynicism and hardness of whatever defences we put up against expressing ourselves in this modern world. I would ask Chuck to bring him with us on the plane to Kenya. He could refuse. But he did not.

We smuggled him across safely and no one was the wiser. Eventually (you always want to know the end of any story) he was transferred to the Jomo Kenyatta hospital in Nairobi where an orthodox above wrist amputation was done under proper anaesthesia.

The Minefield

One of the great annoyances about crowded places is the lack of privacy. I always want a little space for myself and I am sure I share this need with many other people. You do get this space when either in a church or alone in your room. In Loki I was honoured with a room to myself, which was ostensibly a great treat – but I shared it with a wheezy deep freeze that kept buzzing all night and a fridge that burped and groaned intermittently. My room was also the passageway to the communal toilet so that people passed in and out all night assuming that I would neither see nor hear them. To add to this, we kept some stores in my 'bedroom' so that there was no daytime privacy either. I tried to blank out the windows but was conscious that prying eyes peeped in from time to time, not out of malice, but out of curiosity.

From time to time Jim Kenna, an Irish army officer seconded to assist GOAL in logistics, would come up from Nairobi and share my accommodation. Jim was a welcome visitor, not just as a very pleasant companion but also because he would do a 'mossy recko' in the room (mosquito reconnaissance) at least an hour before going to bed.

Kongor was even less private. There was really no place you could go to answer a call of nature. There were curious prying eyes everywhere. And so it happened that I was finished a little earlier than the nurses one afternoon and decided to relieve myself, indeed had to do so, rather urgently. But I wanted privacy. There was nothing for it but to walk into the bush behind the Clinic if I wanted to get out of sight. A small path led into the bush and I slipped off, assuming no one would miss me for a few minutes. I walked along the narrow path, which was bordered by high rushes, and once it made a turn I felt I could safely do my business.

I was hardly finished when I heard shouts from the area of the Clinic and, as I turned to go back, I saw a crowd of people all waving and gesticulating and shouting at me. It took me a few more steps to realise what they were saying. They seemed to be shouting 'Mind ... Mind' which did not make sense until I realised they were shouting 'Mines ... Mines' and were telling me to get off the path. I then made out one voice clearly 'Mines ... mines ... the path is mined'.

I had only 30 yards to walk to safety but they were the longest 30 yards of my life. I stepped off the path and carefully tiptoed on the verge, picking where I would put my foot, knowing that my life (or a limb) depended on it. I ran the last little bit and a great cheer went up from the people. Indeed the whole population of Kongor seemed to have heard of what the mad doctor had done and there was much shaking of heads as well as laughing and backslapping when I finally reached safety.

Evacuate

If Chuck was worried carrying illegals across the border he now became more worried about our own security. Chuck was right. The security situation was rapidly deteriorating,

Government forces were approaching and said to be only a few miles away. On the last trip, he kept the engine of the aeroplane going while it was on the ground and warned us again to drop everything and run to the plane if he sounded the alarm. We had barely finished for the day when we heard him honking the klaxon and, almost immediately afterwards, we heard the sound of gunfire.

People panicked. They ran like rabbits in every direction. The Clinic emptied as if by magic and we could clearly hear Chuck's klaxon now with an urgency that made our pulses race.

And then it started to rain. Not a gentle shower or a ten minutes downpour such as we get at home, but a torrential tropical downpour where you are soaked instantly. Everything was suddenly dark as black clouds blotted out the sun and the whole atmosphere changed to a menacing twilight.

We just upped and ran, heedless of everything except the shape of the plane and Chuck's arms waving frantically at us. One by one we arrived and scrambled on board. A quick count and Chuck took off while one of the nurses banged the back door shut.

As he banked steeply at the end of the grass strip we looked out and could see gun smoke and soldiers crouching and running and darting towards the town. We felt immune in our metal tube but were very sad watching what was happening below, and sadder still when we thought about what would happen when the town fell. Fall it did, later that day, and with that most of the dreams and hopes of the townspeople were dashed to smithereens. Our evacuation was successful but God help those who could not leave. I know they thrashed and ransacked our Clinic but that was not our main concern.

I was only a few months home when I heard that Chuck had died. He was the sole occupant when his plane crashed. I am not sure where it happened but I was very sorry to hear this news for he was a young man and a good man and he will never be forgotten by any of the Goalies he brought in and out of South Sudan in those far off days.

Pretty Petty

You would imagine that living through such hard times and seeing so much sickness, poverty and pain all around would have made us stronger, more caring and more understanding. Not a bit of it. Once safely back in our camp in Loki, we behaved just like any bunch of people thrown into one another's company at home. There were all the usual jealousies, all the real and imagined hurts, all the whispered conversations, all the little cliques and all the petty squabbles over trivial things that you get in any small closed community.

Some were constantly talking about their upcoming R and R and whether they would go to Pemba or Nairobi, or how many days they were due and what expenses they could claim. Others complained that they were assigned more work than the rest, that it always fell to them to clean the common room, that no one ever listened to their problems, that the whole organisation was badly run and that while the top people got well paid they, the real workers, only got a pittance.

Nor did we always treat newcomers properly. I remember an Irish nurse who came out starry eyed and full of zest to work with us, but who was given no specific job to do, was told nothing of the day-to-day running of the mission – much less its aims – and generally she was left alone to 'get on with it'.

I did befriend this girl and we sometimes walked in the desert at evening. She was extremely hurt and disillusioned by everything but most especially by her reception in our Camp.

Yet, individually, our group comprised wonderful people and I do not believe there was anything done or said on purpose to make our welcome to a stranger less than warm. It was just the monotony of life, the hot enervating climate, the lack of privacy in the way we were crowded together, the unending and unwinnable battle against disease, famine and bureaucracy that made us act as we did.

I think you may better understand what I am saying if I mention one small incident. Relations on the ground between GOAL and Concern had become strained, because while GOAL continued to fly into Sudan, Concern had followed the advice of the UN and stopped travelling across the border for security reasons.

This meant that the Concern team had little to do all day while awaiting the security situation to improve. One evening I was asked to dinner by them and I duly went. I forget the dinner but I know it was a pleasant evening and we all enjoyed ourselves. I came home about 10 p.m. and was met by a stony silence from the two Goalies who were still up in our camp. The message was clear. I should not have fraternised with the opposition!

Dreams of Home

The rift was soon mended. Talk at night usually turned to home and a common nostalgia banished any fickle barriers that might have existed between us.

Sometimes after supper, we would join with our Concern friends and together meet up with volunteers from other organisations such as OXFAM or NORAID for a singsong. Some of the Americans sang Stephen Foster songs while the Scandinavians warbled in some ancient Norse tongue.

I would put on a hat and use a cane to take off Maurice Chevalier much to the delight of the onlookers, and this suited me, as I was the eldest of the lot. And there was a small-sized Concern nurse from Dublin who used to sing the *Sally Garden,* so sweetly and so nostalgically, that everyone from all nations hushed and became transported to another gentler world as the notes floated through the tropical night. Some of the Irish sniffled and brushed tears away hoping no one would notice. Of course everyone noticed.

We all went back to normal mundane lives on our return home and got on with things simply by burying the memories of Loki and Kongor deep in our hearts.

CHAPTER 13

BURUNDI, EARLY 1994

This small landlocked country is one of the poorest on earth. Most of its eleven million inhabitants live far below the poverty line and scrape a living from a land that has suffered intensely from climate change and neglect. The three large lakes in the northeast bordering Rwanda and Tanzania are said to have lost half their size by evaporation in the last ten years. Only the majestic lake Tanganyika to the southwest looks as it ever did – deep, still and unfathomable.

Colonists arrived in the late 1800s during the Scramble for Africa. First it was the Germans, then – after World War I (WWI) – the Belgians, and later it became a UN mandated territory. Finally, it became independent in 1962 when it changed its name from Ruanda–Urundi to Burundi.

The ethnic makeup is similar to that in Rwanda: eighty per cent Hutu, fifteen per cent Tutsi and the rest Twa/Pygmy. As in Rwanda, this ethnic division created bitterness, hatred and open violence.

The balance of power continually swung from Hutu to Tutsi and vice versa, and several attempted genocides – by both sides – have been recorded down the years. The 1993 mass killing of Tutsis by Hutus presaged the terrible slaughter in Rwanda the following year, but all along, killing, looting, burnings and rape created a situation where people fled, refugee camps sprang up like mushrooms and the economy descended into ruins.

Even today, despite numerous tentative efforts at power sharing and the solemn declarations of reconciliation and peace – mostly brokered in Arusha – numerous tribal factions and warring groups of renegades and freelancers plague the land, making it one of the most difficult and dangerous places I have ever visited.

From the air, Bujumbura airport looked like a collection of white seashells sparkling in the morning sun. But as we came nearer, the seashells lost their brilliance and looked grey and mottled and neglected. I was not surprised therefore that the arrival's hall was even more neglected, and looking up I could see that the beautifully scalloped domes that we saw from the sky were peppered with holes from a recent mortar attack.

Despite that, the airport officials were smartly dressed in impeccable white uniforms.

Our plane had landed uneventfully and getting through customs and immigration was surprisingly easy, indeed almost casual. There was only a handful of disembarking passengers, most belonging to the UN, which made me the odd man out. My mission was with Concern, which needed a doctor to work with the refugees who were now beginning to flood in from neighbouring countries.

There was less chaos outside the airport than I had expected and I easily got a taxi to take me to the Concern House less than fifteen minutes' away. To get there, we passed through downtown Bujumbura which was also quieter than I expected, but I thought nothing of it at the time. Later I was told that there had been riots the day before I arrived and that an uneasy curfew now existed. I was better off not knowing.

My stay in Bujumbura was short, just a few days, during which the single occupant of the Concern House, a very competent lady, whose name I should remember, made me very welcome and even arranged that the two of us would drive to the Lake on the following Sunday and have a swim.

Although most of Burundi is quite elevated and mosquitoes are scarce, nonetheless, it has an oppressive equatorial climate and the thought of a swim in Lake Tanganyika sounded most attractive.

A Swim in Lake Tanganyika

Lake Tanganyika is the longest and the second deepest fresh-water lake in the world. It is older than Lake Malawi, but unlike the latter, it is free of bilharzia. This is probably due to turbulent winds that make life difficult for infected snails to transmit the disease to humans. I knew this at the time and so the prospect of cooling off in the pristine waters of Lake Tanganyika appealed to me greatly.

We had attended ten o'clock Mass in a nearby church and once again I was thrilled by the rhythmic beating of drums, the harmonious spontaneous singing and the general colour so typical of Mass in Africa. It was warm and getting warmer as the Mass went on, especially as the sermon seemed interminable. People fanned themselves with anything they could find and some left and returned obviously hoping that the priest had finished his harangue. At the Sign of Peace, there was general commotion. Everyone wanted to shake hands with or embrace everyone else, and it was several minutes before things settled down. After a full two hours, the Mass was finally over and we all dispersed into the sunshine. Even still no one was in a hurry, least of all the priest.

Immediately afterwards, we set off for the lake, just the two of us, with our packed lunch, towels and swimming togs. It was a beautiful day. A soft breeze cooled us as we drove out of the city and on to the narrow winding road that skirts the lake. The lake was on our right and there was a high rocky escarpment on our left. This was surely a geologist's delight, with all kinds of different strata clearly visible in the rock face. Had we driven far enough and veered inland, we would have reached the Ruvyirona River, believed by many to be the *really true* source of the Nile – despite competitors in Rwanda and Uganda. Had we gone north instead of south we might have met the baby crocodile who later turned into a notorious man eater named Gustave! So south was a good choice.

However, we had not gone more than a few miles when we were stopped by soldiers who said we could not go further. No reason was given nor did we ask. They were curious but polite and none of them looked for money.

We duly turned around and, after making a ten-point turn on the narrow road, found a small grass patch recessed between two rocky outcrops – a perfect picnic spot. It was half in the shade and half in the sun, ideal for our purposes. We lay in the sunny part for a little while but, having no books to read and no radio to listen to, we quickly decided to swim and then eat lunch.

I remember that the water was clear and limpid and, most of all, freezing cold. So cold in fact that neither of us stayed in more than a few minutes. Yet we both frolicked in the water like school children before climbing out and letting the sun warm up our shocked bodies.

Coke and homemade sandwiches never tasted better. There is something magical about eating *al fresco* that transforms ordinary food into *haute cuisine*. I am sure that part of this magic is due to being young and hungry.

Afterwards, we lay there soaking up the sun and listening to the gentle lapping of water on the rocky shore.

By mutual consent, we stirred ourselves when the sun started to dip and made for home while there was still plenty of light. I know I slept well, even though my mattress was lumpy, the electricity was off and the plumbing noisy enough to wake *Rip van Winkle*.

The house was ransacked a few days later but I had left for up country so only heard the news by chance. Everything was taken, even the light bulbs. Luckily, no one was in the house at the time and so no one was hurt.

Exploding Lakes

You probably never heard of exploding lakes? These are lakes, based on volcanoes, which erupt from time to time, emitting vast amounts of CO_2 gas. The surrounding countryside is bathed in the deadly gas at concentrations sufficient to kill people. This happened in the Cameroun in 1984 when Lake Monoun exploded. When Lake Nyos – also in the Cameroun – exploded two years later, thirty-seven people died and a deadly cloud of CO_2 suffocated almost 2,000 locals.

Lake Tanganyika is a likely candidate to explode any time. Happily it was fast asleep 25 years ago, when we dived into it.

Kirundo

I saw little of Bujumbura as my transport to Kirundo, a town in the north of the country near the Rwandan border, came sooner than expected. Médecins sans Frontières (MSF) were going in convoy to Kirundo and obliged me with a free ride. My memories of the 225 km journey are of driving through rolling hills, lush farmland, patchy tea and banana plantations and numerous small villages. But of danger, we saw none. I was dropped off outside our house on the outskirts of Kirundo, a short walk from Lake Rwihinda, known locally as the 'lake of birds'.

There were several other volunteers in the house and they told me that things were quiet just then, but that thousands of refugees were on the way not only from Rwanda but also from other parts of Burundi and even the Congo. Our team was earmarked to set up a camp for them and run it as best as we could. There was little I could do until the refugees arrived.

For several days, I did nothing but eat, read and sleep. Each morning, I would walk down to the lake and watch the birth of a new beautiful dawn and thrill to the sight of the sun rising majestically over the lake. Each evening, I would return and marvel at the flocks of birds careering and wheeling in the sky, as they made their way home for the night. Many settled down in a small island that is now protected as a natural aviary, others settled in the branches of trees nearer the shore. All filled the evening air with different melodies and there is no doubt that they had picked one of the most beautiful places on earth to make their home.

By now I was fretful and weary doing nothing, so I volunteered to help prepare sites and set up tents for the influx of refugees that we expected any day.

To do this, we had to acquire a piece of land that was near a water supply. Our field Director liaised with the local administration to identify and lease a suitable site. Then engineers from another NGO came and sank a few wells and started on sanitation and drainage works. Others came and organised water tankers from Kirundo and promised deliveries of food once a month. Locals were employed to dig trenches for communal toilets. A little town was taking shape.

I hated measuring out plots of land for each refugee family. We had to adhere to the minimum size for each plot as recommended by the WHO and each one had to be roped off securely. The terrain was bumpy, the grasses were long and the insect bites and bramble scratches were many. I would be glad when the refugees began to arrive. I could then revert to far easier medical work.

Meantime, apart from measuring out plots and setting up tents, I was given the job of sourcing ropes and buying rice, sorghum and manioc so that we could feed the refugees until the UN took over regular food supplies. I know I made poor bargains but I figured the locals should not be denied a small windfall in the midst of all the misery.

Warriors with Spears

There was an MSF facility not far away and during a quiet time, I went to them offering my services until the refugees arrived. I was in their Clinic one afternoon when two of their nurses who had been doing outreach clinic told me this story. How true or exaggerated it is I am not sure but I tell it anyway.

One afternoon, after a particularly hot and busy day in a bush clinic, they decided to take a short-cut home. This meant driving the jeep across scrubland rather than taking the longer route by a road.

They were half way across when suddenly a group of twenty yelling African warriors appeared. They were wearing only lion cloths and had white streaks painted on their faces, which made them look fearsome. They were charging wildly at a retreating band of young men who were fleeing for their lives. The attackers had spears, which they flourished about menacingly, but it was the yelling that was the scariest.

The MSF nurses did not wait to see what would happen. They screamed at their driver to get out fast *Vite…Vite* …. He needed no encouragement. The Toyota bounded ahead in a cloud of dust that must have dampened the ardour of the attackers – at least momentarily. I like to think that how they gave enough time for their prey to escape.

Nowadays, the nurses would have taken a video with their cell phones and sold it to a TV station.

The Refugees Arrive

They started as a trickle and finished as a flood. Most were fleeing Rwanda although some had come from further afield, from the Congo and Sudan. Ultimately they merged into one amorphous mass of people, lost, homeless and destitute. My memories. Mankind on the move. Struggling, weary and carrying pathetic loads on their backs. What agonies they carried inside themselves no one will ever know.

Even the kindest person eventually becomes desensitised to the suffering of others. That is a fact. I hope it never happens to me but I also know that you have to develop a kind of hardness if you are to maintain law and order and stop the strong ones pushing the weaker ones aside. As a medic it is easy to tend to wounds, dole out medicine and set up drips on the very sick. It is much harder as a human to share mentally in the suffering of one's fellow man.

Ghosts

Perhaps the strain of the work, perhaps the constant bustle and noise of the day, perhaps even the sun, made us all a little giddy in the evenings when we got 'home' and indulged in a warm beer or two.

I must have been in such a mood one evening when one of the group started telling ghost stories. We were five or six of us, a mixed bunch of nurses, a maintenance man and myself, all slouched in chairs and bean bags, with just a bush lamp for light. It cast long flickering shadows that danced on the walls and gave an eerie glow to our pale white faces.

I think the nurse who started the conversation about ghosts was from Co Tipperary but I cannot be sure. She was obviously enjoying telling us about some headless horseman that her grandfather swore he saw riding along the country byways near his cottage one moonlit night. Others joined in with their stories once she had finished and always there was a pause before someone else took up the theme.

My contribution was weak but they all pretended to be spellbound as I told them of the haunted house I had seen in my childhood. It was a solitary house standing bleakly on a stretch of road between Passage East and Woodstown in Co. Waterford. It had been deserted for many years. It was deserted since no one would buy it because of 'unnatural goings on' there at night. People passing the house on a dark night would hear sounds, like the crying of a child. Perhaps a child had died there? Perhaps an unwanted baby had been strangled there? No one knew. But many heard the crying and moreover many saw the top windows glow with a strange light.

My mother, in her usual pragmatic way, had told us children that such tales were usually reported by tipsy farmers going home from the pub in the early hours of the morning. She may have been right. But I did not want to spoil my story with any earthly explanation and so my listeners – and myself – shivered fearfully at the thought of a little dead baby calling for help night after night.

Our evening ended on a lighter note. I told them the purportedly true story of a hunchback who died in the West of Ireland many years ago. I believe it was somewhere in the area of Headford that this occurred, but I may be wrong.

The mourners were having the usual all-night wake in the hunchback's house and were enjoying plenty of drink, lots of thick ham sandwiches and an ample supply of homemade fruit cake supplied by the neighbours.

As was the custom – and still is in many rural parts of Ireland – local men dug the grave and the local women laid out the dead and prepared the food.

But how could they lay out a hunchback? The solution was found by two of his cousins who placed him on the kitchen table, forcibly straightened his back and secured his legs and arms to the stout wooden legs of the table with ropes. The ropes were hidden by cloths, but not completely, for the hunchback's inquisitive cat has pulled at one corner exposing a section of rope beneath.

All the rosaries had been said, and anyway everyone was sure the hunchback was now in Heaven, so that more prayers would be superfluous. If he was in Hell then of course prayers would be pointless. In either case, it was time to drink to the dead man's health and drink generously, for he was truly 'a dacent poor crátúr'. Everyone, be he saint or scoundrel, is 'a dacent poor crátúr' when dead.

Midnight was fast approaching and the merriment increased by the minute. At the stroke of twelve on the dresser clock, the hunchback sprang up from the table and sat there glaring at everyone just as he did when he was alive.

The mourners – well 'under the weather' with drink – now panicked and made for the kitchen door and off out into the darkness, invoking the Lord and every saint they could think of as they scattered in all directions.

Only the two cousins and the hunchback remained behind, all three now bent double with laughter. That is except for the hunchback. He was dead all right, and certainly not laughing. But the two cousins were very much alive and toasting each other liberally with *poitín*.

'Boy of boy, t'was aisey scare them after all...' chuckled cousin no. 1.

'Shure I thought we'd never cut through them ropes in time….' replied cousin no. 2, gulping another slug from the bottle.

'Will we straighten him out again?'

'No, leave him alone. T'was good enough he looked all bent in half when he was alive. T'will do him powerful now in the next world'

'Did we do a sin?'

"Ah, shush your gob….'

No one had noticed the pair cutting the ropes.

'Time for bed' I announced, breaking the atmosphere of unreality that had descended on the group.

One-by-one we got up, each going his or her own way, reluctantly breaking the cosy atmosphere of childhood reveries. I remained in the room for a little, just sitting there in the dark, alone and strangely content.

The house we were lodged in must have been some kind of hostel at one time because it consisted of an action area in front (hall, sitting room and kitchen) and a sleeping area behind (bedrooms and toilets). The bedroom windows overlooked a sloping lawn, which had been neglected for years and in which the grass was now a series of mottled yellowish clumps. There were eight bedrooms in all.

By now the house was silent apart from the comforting tick tock of a wag-on-the-wall clock over the archway that led to the bedroom corridor. I reckoned everyone was in bed, dog tired after another hot day and now ready for sleep. Probably already dreaming of ghosts and spirits and strange things that go bump in the night.

I crept silently to my room and pulled the white linen sheet off my bed. I located my torch on the bedside table and noiselessly slipped out and down the corridor again.

I opened the front door as quietly as I could and made my way to the centre of the lawn where I could be seen from all of the bedroom windows. I now put the sheet over my head and held the torch between it and my face.

Once in position I switched on the torch so that my face would look frightening and then, since no one came to any window, I began a low moaning.

I think, *I hope,* I fooled people for a moment. Windows opened and faces appeared as I began to approach the building in a swaying motion. Unfortunately, the sheet did not reach the ground and my legs were visible from below my knees.

'Oh go to bed' I heard someone shout. 'Dom ... Stop fooling around ... For goodness sake ... we can't get a wink of sleep....' Other less polite phrases were hurled at me and then humiliated and feeling foolish, I stumbled and almost fell. This was greeted with whoops of laughter and the sound of closing windows.

There was nothing for it but to return to the house and go to my room. My joke had fallen flat that night but remained a topic of amused conversation for some time afterwards.

Seriously, I do not know what made me behave so foolishly.

I slept to the sound of Mary Black singing something about a woman's love. One of the nurses kept playing a cassette of Mary Blacks songs repeatedly in the Land Rover on our way to the Refugee Camp. Now I was getting it by night as well as by day.

CHAPTER 14

DARK DAYS IN RWANDA
1994–1995

The Land

Rwanda, like Burundi, is one of several small landlocked countries situated in the middle of Africa. It is a fertile hilly place bathed in deep lush green vegetation and dense rain forests. The rains feed many lakes, which, though small in comparison to Lake Victoria, are large by European standards. Most are teeming with fish and so provide lots of nourishment for the local population.

The steep hills of Rwanda are ridged to prevent the rain from washing away the soil and are farmed almost to their tops. The lowlands provide ideal pasture for cattle and for the cultivation of cereals. Rice grows well in the rich moist marshlands of the valleys and, although only started in 1950, rice is now one of the most important sectors of Rwanda's agriculture.

Rwanda has been compared to Switzerland regarding both its terrain and hard-working people. This is a fair comparison. You will find alpine flowers, deep glaciers and snow-capped peaks in Rwanda's Rwenzori Mountains just as in Switzerland. But you will come across giant lobelias and exotic wildlife, which you will not find in Switzerland or anywhere else in Europe. In addition, Rwanda is a host to the Mountain Gorillas, a must see for any traveller to East Africa.

However, while on the surface, life has a gentler pace than Switzerland, the majority of people have little of this worlds goods and the average farmer subsists on farming just 1 hectare of land.

Before the genocide, over seven million people lived in Rwanda. After the genocide, the population had fallen to just five million and most people's wealth was wiped out. Switzerland supports 8.3 million, virtually all in comfort.

The average person living in the West had never heard of Rwanda until 1994. Some were familiar with a country in the African Great lake region called Ruanda-Urundi but in 1962 this had been split into the new states of Rwanda and Burundi and, like all name changes, it took many years for the new names to come into common usage. Those who had heard of Rwanda associated it with Dian Fossey and the Mountain Gorillas, but that was about the extent of their knowledge.

The genocide changed all that. In 1994 and 1995, the appalling happenings in Rwanda became the major media topic throughout the world.

I dare not compete with all that has been written about the cause of the genocide but a little background to the most brutal holocaust since the Nazi concentration camps is necessary if what I say is to make any sense.

Tutsi–Hutu Antagonism

Probably uniquely in Africa, the borders of Rwanda predated colonial times. And so that country was always an entity that stood on its own and in which the inhabitants were never subjected to slavery. However, intertribal and inter-communal strife was always a feature of life, and this discord held development back for generations.

Outsiders lumped the different tribes together calling them all the Banyarwanda people. But they were not homogenous. As in Burundi, eighty four per cent were Hutu, fifteen per cent were Tutsi and the remaining one per cent were Twa (pygmy people).

The Tutsis, like the Jews in Europe, the Igbos in Nigeria and the Asians in Uganda, felt they would be squashed out unless they worked harder than the Hutus. Thus, they stuck together, supported one another and favoured the advancement of their own kind over anyone else. Ultimately, the Tutsis held most positions of authority, were the better-educated and controlled commerce in the region. I expect they saw themselves as superior to either the Hutu or Twa who looked at them with an envy bordering on hatred.

It is understandable then, that even in pre-colonial times, there were regular violent confrontations between the Tutsis and the Hutus.

The European powers made things worse. In 1884, the Germans came and forcibly established themselves when creating German East Africa (Rwanda, Burundi and Tanganyika). They later institutionalised tribal antagonism by issuing separate identity cards to everyone, based – extraordinarily – on nose and facial measurements.

Four types were identified: Hutu, Tutsi, Twa and the Naturalised. This fitted in nicely with the wave of fascism then sweeping Europe. Unfortunately, these cards would provide an easy way of identifying who should be slaughtered 50 years later.

Things even got worse after WWI when the Belgians came. They continued the German policy of giving preferment to Tutsis over Hutus by appointing Tutsis to the majority of senior administrative, professional and technological posts. This fuelled further resentment in the numerically superior

Hutus of Ruanda-Urundi who now found an unlikely ally in the powerful Catholic Church.

The Catholic Church had been opposed to the introduction of tribal identity cards in 1935. It recognised that this facilitated segregation based on one's tribal origin. Nowhere was this more apparent than in education where overt discrimination clearly favoured the Tutsi. Since the Church ran and funded many schools, it was in a position to change this and so by the time of Independence in 1962, the Church had provided education for many Hutus.

A by-product of this, probably an intended dividend, was the entry of many young Hutu men and women into seminaries and convents.

A new generation of highly educated articulate Hutu had emerged. Many got jobs in the media and expressed their outrage at the way Hutus had been repressed for generations. Some radical populist elements went further and actively incited violence to redress injustice. However, the majority knew that in time a fairer distribution of jobs and wealth was inevitable and so, whatever their inner thoughts, they remained on good terms with their Tutsi neighbours and wanted only peace and prosperity for all Rwandans.

Unfortunately, the extreme elements won out – as usual. The aggrieved, militant and semi-educated Hutus who demanded immediate action successfully initiated recurring pogroms that resulted in more and more Tutsis fleeing to neighbouring countries.

By 1990, the scene was set for an explosion of some sort.

In that year exiled Tutsis, loosely grouped as the Rwandan Patriotic Front (RPF), invaded Rwanda, and although they were unsuccessful in 'reconquering' the country, they greatly undermined the power of the moderate Hutu President, Juvénal Habyarimana. Indeed, the invasion made things worse, for it had pushed Rwanda into a *de facto* civil war.

Juvénal Habyarimana, who had changed from an earlier policy of militant extremism to one of inclusion and toleration, was appalled. He wanted peace. Accordingly, he compromised by agreeing to a power-sharing government in what became known as the *Arusha Accord*.

But this satisfied neither side. 'Hutu Power' dominated the airwaves and each violent act resulted in a reprisal and in further violence.

Genocide Looms

Matters came to a head on 6 April 1994 when the airplane carrying Habyarimana and Burundian President Cyprien Ntaryamira (also a Hutu) was shot down as it descended into Kigali airport. Everyone on board was lost. The weight of evidence provided by French investigators later suggested that this was done by Hutu extremists who wanted to get rid of their moderate President and who wanted to embark on a Hitler-like 'final solution' for the 'Tutsi problem'.

Over the previous years, Hutus had been given machetés and more recently automatic weapons imported from Egypt, so most observers now believe that the genocide that followed the downing of the presidential aircraft had been planned for a long time.bjk

The 100-Day Butchery: April 1994

The butchery began the day after the presidential plane was shot down and lasted unabated for the next 100 days. The military, the police and a loose lawless militia, the *interahamwe* (lit. 'those who stick together'), erected barricades and killed everyone who had a non-Hutu identity card. Tutsis and moderate Hutus were hacked to death. Thousands were rounded up and mass murdered; those found fleeing were driven down by lorries and cars as they fled and their bodies thrown into the river or simply left to rot.

By July, 800,000 Rwandans, mostly Tutsis, were dead, and all Tutsi homes were destroyed, looted or occupied by Hutus.

Wicked Women

Women joined in the massacres and several, including the notorious Angéline Mukandutiye, a director of primary schools in Kigali, directed killer squads to eliminate 'the snakes' and 'the cockroaches'. A Benedictine nun, Sister Julienne Kizito, who became later known as the 'Animal', was seen to actively pass cans of petrol to militia who were dousing and burning their victims alive. She later escaped to Belgium. Another woman, a laywoman, Odette Uwimana, was known as 'Satan' for the way she treated anyone in her clutches. Strangely enough she was still working in a Parish in Kigali when I was there on a second visit in 1995.

But possibly the most brutal of all the women who took part in the genocide was Rose Karushara the 'butcher of Kimisagara'. No book could contain a list of all the savageries she perpetrated without burning itself for shame.

Many well-educated women politicians, journalists, teachers, doctors, nurses and administrators actively supported the killings and even school children got caught up in an ululating frenzy of slaughter.

Some used the word 'Ndabaga' to describe the actions of women killers during the genocide. The word Ndabaga is used in Rwanda to describe heroic means, especially by women, in desperate situations. They debase that name. Ndabaga was a revered young woman who took up arms many years ago and defeated an enemy who had killed all the men folk in her village. She was a Rwandan Joan of Arc.

Madame Agathe

One of the many atrocities that received worldwide attention was the assassination of Agathe Uwilingiyimana, ('Madame Agathe'). She was a popular figure, and much loved by everyone, including President Juvénal.

At 9 a.m. on 7 April 1994, a blood-crazed Presidential Guard shot both her and her husband while their children hid behind furniture. The world stood aghast. And did nothing. Agathe was 40 years old.

A small force called United Nations Assistance Mission in Rwanda had been set up in October 1993 in response to worldwide concern at the persecution of Tutsis and of moderate Hutus and, while their mandate was chiefly a monitoring one, a special detachment had been sent to protect Madame Agathe.

Shamefully they complied with orders and laid down their weapons at the feet of the Presidential Guard allowing the assassination of her and her husband to go ahead unimpeded. Ten Belgian soldiers were then taken to Kigali Military Barracks where they were tortured and executed. The madness went unabated and still the world stood still, waiting and watching and talking, talking and talking. Same is happening in Syria while I write these lines.

The film *Hotel Rwanda* captures the eerie, dark, surrealistic atmosphere of those days. But even that film, moving as it was, cannot begin to convey the real story. How can any film re-enact atrocities such as those which took place in Ntrama church where over 5,000 people seeking refuge were 'killed by grenade, machete, rifle or burnt alive?'

The stench of bodies, the screams of children and the howls of blood-hungry mobs should remain forever fixed in the annals of the mankind. Could mankind but remember them.

The Twa

I think it is important to mention the fate of the Twa pygmies. No one bothers to talk about them; it is as if they were not important, did not exist. The genocide represented the peak of a suffering for these people that had gone on over the years. Any Twa who had a home was now either killed or driven into the forests where many died of fever and starvation. Those who had no homes ran to the bush and God knows where they are now.

Some remained and some crept back. You can see them surviving as beggars on the streets of Kigali today.

June–July 1994: UN Shame

It was June before the UN responded in any meaningful way to stop the killing. Their intervention was called *Operation Turquoise* and involved the deployment of 2,500 French soldiers. This slowed the slaughter but its effectiveness was more apparent than real and actually made things worse for many.

Large numbers of people, mainly Tutsi, now felt safe to return, thinking that at last they could come out from hiding. Most never reached their homes, for the Hutu army and militia was waiting for them and the slaughter recommenced.

It seems incredible that this could have happened under the noses of the UN troops. More incredible still is the fact that a similar situation occurred in Srebrenica exactly two years later when 8,000 Bosniaks were mown down, while the UN mandated Dutchbat (Dutch battalion) stood by, again unable to intervene because they were there as a peace-observers rather than peace-enforcers.

Eventually, an invading Tutsi force, the RPF, put an end to the killing. They took Kigali on 4th July and reconquered the whole of Rwanda a few weeks later. The national gendarmerie and the dreaded government-backed militias, including the *Interahamwe* and *Impuzamugambi*, were disbanded, resulting in a huge exodus of Hutus. Revenge was in the air.

Many innocent people were slaughtered by the RPF, among them were the Archbishop of Kigali and two bishops and thirteen priests in Kabgayi, merely because they were *suspected* of backing the genocide. I think their failure to condemn the killings outright was due to their fear that all priests and sisters would become a target.

Which does not excuse their comparative silence. See too how the French forces looked on in pain, but held to their avowed stance of staying 'neutral'.

Both the guilty and innocent now fled for fear of reprisals and most of them found some kind of precarious shelter in Goma. Goma lies just across the border in the DCR, then Zaire.

Goma camp was soon to become synonymous with disease, torture, rape and bloodshed.

Robert Kajuga

In one of the inexplicable ironies of history, Jerry Robert Kajuga, President of the *Interahamwe,* one of the most feared and most vicious paramilitary groups involved in the genocide of the Tutsis, was himself a Tutsi! His family had acquired Hutu identity papers thus hiding their Tutsi origins. When he realised that the RPF could not be stopped, he fled to the Congo posing as a Hutu. He found refuge there for a few years but was always in fear for his life. He looked around for someplace safe and slipped away quietly, this time to South Sudan. Here he was warmly received – at first. But politics prevailed, and later, probably because South Sudan needed international recognition, he was arrested by UN security forces and deported back to Kigali.

He was tried in Arusha in Tanzania and convicted of complicity in genocide. He is currently serving a life sentence in Rwanda.

I think the treatment of Kajuga by the present Rwandan regime is a shining example of how a civilised society uses the rule of justice rather than the rule of revenge.

I have tried to condense a most complicated and convoluted piece of history into a few paragraphs. In doing so I am sure I have given a picture that is neither fair nor comprehensive. For this I ask indulgence. I also apologise for the difficult names. And if I have given the impression that the genocide was a simple Hutu versus Tutsi affair then I mislead. Many moderate Hutus were slaughtered and many moderate Hutus hid Tutsis at great peril to their own lives.

The Church too gave sanctuary to many thousands of people and it was an exceptional nun or priest who turned anyone away.

Rwanda: Personal Experiences
The Devil Dances, Demons Delight and Darkness Descends Over the Land

Like many thousands of people all over the world I was moved to pity, shame and anger by the unfolding massacre shown nightly on our TV screens from April to July 1994. It is little wonder that I should have set off to Rwanda with a team of nurses as soon as I could; yet it was August before I got there. I was a director of Refugee Trust at the time (now renamed Vita) and so was the obvious choice to lead our medical team. Others did the logistical work and our immediate coordinator was Ann Malone, a teacher from Greystones, Co Wicklow. Ann was a capable and determined young woman meticulous in her methods and uncompromising in her dedication to do her best.

Our medical team consisted of just four nurses and myself. All four – Brenda, Finola, Dorothea and Eileen – were religious sisters and all were free to travel at short notice. Later, in succeeding visits, we recruited lay nurses so that our group became more representative of all strands of Irish society.

Since it was impossible for us to fly to Kigali, we first landed in Entebbe, Uganda. Here the happenings in Rwanda made a direct impact, not just because of the refugees who were streaming across the border but also because of the large numbers of dead Tutsis who had been washed up on the shores of Lake Victoria. This horrified the Ugandans who saw it as an affront to God.

The Rivers of Death

The bodies that they saw were usually mutilated, sometimes half decomposed and sometimes half eaten by crocodiles. All were grotesquely swollen. Most had been dumped – living and dead, young and old – into the Nyabarongo and Ruvabu rivers in Rwanda. From here, they floated down the Kagera river through Burundi before issuing into the west side of Lake Victoria near the Tanzanian town of Bukoba. Finally, they were deposited ashore in Uganda. Some say the rivers ran red with Tutsi blood. One witness described the way bodies were dumped into the Nyabarongo River as 'paper is thrown into the dustbin' (Africa Rights, 1995: 111). The lucky ones who escaped the river fled to Tanzania across the Rusumo Bridge, which spans the Kagera near the famous Rusumo Falls. Over a quarter of a million people fled across the Rusumo Bridge on 28/29 of April 1994, in the fastest and largest race for safety ever recorded by the UN.

August 1994

By the time I arrived in August 1994, the mass killings were virtually finished. Yet several bodies were caught up in reeds on the riverbank and made fine food for predators as they lay there unshriven and unmourned. All their relations were now either dead or missing. This is true.

Some say that those rivers of death constitute yet another source of the Nile, but such considerations did not trouble us as we drove across Uganda and crossed the equator, just north of Masaka, so familiar to me from previous visits to Uganda. We ended up in the town of Kabale near the Rwandan border.

Here we stayed in the Victoria Guest House, which was close to the centre of the town, but was nonetheless in a quiet and relatively safe location. Our plan was to rehabilitate the Health Complex in Ruhengeri in the northwest of Rwanda. It was one of the last places to be liberated by the Rwanda Patriotic Army (RPA), the armed branch of the RPF. Of course, like all 'liberations', this one was sullied by revenge and reprisals against Hutus – many of whom were innocent of any crime.

Ironically, the RPA of 1994 would turn against the democratically elected government of Rwanda in 2000, and was only thwarted in its efforts to take Kigali when French and Congolese forces came to the aid of loyal Rwandan troops. History is full of ironies, paradoxes and unpredictable twists and turns.

The Victoria Guest House was shaped like a rectangle with an open front. The guest rooms occupied the two larger arms. The room furnishings were sparse; the beds hard, the mosquito nets full of holes and there were no locks on the ill-fitting doors. But it was home, and we were happy to have a room each where we could cut out the happenings of the day and be alone.

We knew little of the historical complexities of Rwanda as we bunked down for our first night in our new lodgings. It was good to have arrived and we were determined to do our best even if our best was to fall short of what was needed.

The morning after we arrived, we drove the few miles to Rwanda, crossed the border without any problem and made the twenty miles or so to Kigali where we had to register with the Ministry for Immigration. We had armed guards to protect us but none of us were sure what they would do if confronted by real danger.

The journey to Kigali was eerie. The excellent tarred road to the capital was completely empty. There was none of the usual traffic one expects on African roads. There were no colour-ful 'mammy wagons' crammed with passengers and loaded with crates and boxes. There were no big black 'high nellies' wobbling along, laden with impossible loads of bananas or charcoal on back and front and carrying a passenger or two on the cross bar. There were no streams of people bearing huge loads on their heads, going to market or visiting neighbours.

The countryside looked sad, as if in sympathy with the people. The sides of the road were empty, bereft of all life. Yes, there was the occasional sighting of a woman or a child in the distance, but they left the road as soon as they became aware of our approach. Was it fear? Was it guilt? Who knows?

Kigali itself was not much better. There were some stalls on the side of the road as one approached the centre of the city just before the roundabout that leads to the *Mille Colline*, the hotel on the hill made famous in *Hotel Rwanda*. There were even some traders selling little African carvings and other souvenirs as one approached the hotel. The buyers were mainly EU personnel or foreign UN peacekeepers. There was no electricity and the water and sewage system was malfunctioning to say the least.

Yet there was life behind closed doors. Black market racketeers touted their wares and beckoned us in. Money exchangers were standing at corners offering a fabulous rate of local currency in exchange for US dollars. Anything and everything was for sale at a bargain price.

Yes, there is resilience in human nature that is simply amazing. I'm sure we Irish had it in the great famine of 1847–1849. Londoners showed it during the blitz of WWII, Jews showed it in Hitler's concentration camps, Germans showed it in 1945 in the ruins of Berlin, the Japanese had it after Hiroshima and Nagasaki and the Rwandans had it in 1994. Adversity definitely brings out the best in most of us.

My own contribution was little and this is not false modesty. I travelled in the back of an open pick-up with the rest of our team each morning across the border from Uganda and went home each evening, leaving work about 4 p.m. We distributed food and clothes to as many as we could.

We employed locals to rebuild and refurbish the Health Centre that was not actually at Ruhengeri, but in Kiyanza, several miles east of Ruhengeri and off the main road. This involved travelling up a very steep hill to finally get there. It was difficult to access, even with our four-wheel drive, and virtually impossible for normal traffic other than oxen. There used to be a 'medical' bus that transported patients to and from the Centre but this was now a burned out skeleton, rather like a dead whale lying on a beach, with its metal ribs exposed to the scorching sun.

When we finally arrived Laurencie and Pascalie, two of the surviving Health Centre attendants, met us. All the rest had either been murdered or had fled. They were excited to see us and so grateful for anything we did for them.

I remember Laurencie well. She was pregnant and was clearly not too far from delivery date.

I doled out medicine, delivered a few babies, tried to organise the clinics, helped register patients and gave a hand with distributing food and medicines. There was nothing heroic in my work. Each night I slept well in the comparative comfort of the Victoria Guest house in Kabale and gradually we all fell into a comfortable routine. Yet we knew we should be based in Rwanda for as time passed, border crossings became more difficult, officials became more officious, and the RPA soldiers more arrogant and even threatening.

So we were all relieved when we found accommodation in the *San Famille* convent in Kigali, which was conveniently situated close to the centre of town and the roundabout that leads to the *Mille Colline*. There was not much privacy since we slept in cubicles reminiscent of boarding school days, but it was so much more central and so much easier to travel to and from work each day. The convent is in the same compound as St Pauls Church and hostel, making it an ideal location for the less wealthy traveller even today.

We did not really get to know the Sisters in the convent but gathered that at least 12 of them had been murdered in the genocide. One evening, a police wagon drove to the front door and demanded to see one of the remaining Sisters. She was dragged out and taken away, presumably to be shot. I do not know if she was a Hutu or a Tutsi – or either. Maybe she had been a collaborator in the genocide or maybe she had hidden somebody. Whatever the cause of her abduction, there was a palpable gloom after she had gone and no one seemed happy to talk about it.

In the following months, I made three trips to Rwanda all of differing lengths from three months to one month. They almost blend into one experience now that over twenty years have passed. Mostly my time there was uneventful and the work repetitive and hum drum. The heart had been torn out of a people who had lost all zest for life.

After a While

After a while, you become used to working with few medicines and little help. After a while, you become used to going to the ICRC or the EU missions and begging for food, materials or money. And after a while, you get used to being refused or put off with plausible excuses. After a while, you even get used to seeing sickness, poverty and death all around and you get used to hearing stories of murder, rape and pillage that should make you scream in anger.

After a while, you get used to Hell.

So it is the little things that I now remember, the little things, just that bit out of the ordinary. For example, by pure chance, on one occasion, my car refused to go up the steep hill that led to the Health Centre. The engine just died. I was at the foot of the hill and there was nothing I could do but get out and wait on the side of the road hoping that assistance would come sooner than later.

This was morning time and it was pleasant to sit on a rock and let the sun warm me as I watched the busy streams of ants scamper about between the stones at my feet. Ants are so orderly and so positive in their movements that no matter what obstacle they encounter they seem unfazed and just make their way around it. I whiled away the time putting little pebbles in their path and watching them march around them or I would block their way completely – as I thought – with a large stone, but somehow they would find a way over or else squeeze under it through the only spot where the stone did not lie quite flat on the ground.

If I were in a similar situation in Europe, I would be phoning the AA, or the police would make me push the car off the road or I would find that all my efforts to hail down a passing vehicle were in vain. Not so in Africa. I knew that the first person who came along would stop to help and so I sat there without a worry in the world.

Sure enough, after about an hour, an elderly man came into view pushing his bike, which was laden with what seemed to me like the whole contents of his house. Perhaps it was.

He could not speak either English or French but he immediately knew I was in trouble. He grinned showing an edentulous mouth apart from one or two yellow stubs. He waved his arms in a gesture that I hoped meant he would go for help. I thanked him as best I could and we both parted with many nods of the head and lots of vain pointing to the now silent engine of the car. Within a short time one, then two, then a sizeable crowd of people appeared from nowhere.

They all looked thin and miserable compared to this one well-fed white man, but they were all good humoured and set to the task of pushing the car up the steep incline with gusto. Meantime I had got into the car, put it in gear and hey presto, as the car gained momentum, the engine sprang to life and off I went. Normally, one would do this going down an incline. I had done it going up an incline.

In gratitude, I stopped on the first flat piece of road and waited for my friends to catch up while I kept the engine running. They came up to me all smiles and I thanked them as I always did by giving them money. Everyone got a single dollar bill.

People condemn the practise of giving money directly in this fashion. 'It makes them dependent', 'it creates a hand-out mentality' and 'it spoils them'. I understand what they are saying but I understand better the desperate poverty in which so many people live and *I know* that hard cash is the only thing that can immediately make life just a little bit easier.

Of course, it is temporary and of course it can be called condescending, but it is the one commodity that a poor person can use to buy what he needs most, be it food, clothes or fees to send a child to school. Even in the worst places that I have been, hard cash can buy the necessities of life. Everything is there if you have the money to pay for it. That is why I bring a couple of hundred dollars in single notes whenever I travel to a place where I know that a dollar a day is as much as you can earn if you are lucky enough to get work – and be paid.

One of the group, a little older than the rest, spoke to me in English.

'Thank you sir, we know you are the doctor come here to help our people.

These are hard times'

'I wish I could do more to help.' Then to make conversation I asked, 'How is life for you now?'

'It is bad. Not as bad as before with the killings, but bad... bad. We could not plant crops during the war ... many ... so many people were murdered or carried away or have fled. Only old men and young children are left, most of the youth has gone....' His voice trailed off.

There was sadness about him as if all the light had gone out of his life.

'And there is not enough food now?' A rather stupid question.

'No, we have little money to buy food and no food of our own. These are bad, bad times....' He repeated once more.

Mostly I have difficulty in making small decisions. For example, if I am out shopping, I find it difficult to choose which type of butter to buy or which brand of ketchup, or even which queue to join (usually the shortest which turns out to be short because it is the slowest). But when I am moved by a strong emotion, such as I was that day, I have no difficulty in making a choice even if I am sorry the moment I have opened my big mouth.

'I will get you food, I promise.'

And then, he did something that always embarrasses me. He knelt down and kissed the back of my hands. Oh God, I felt awful. I honestly believe, with every fibre of my being, in the equality of all human beings and hold that the dignity of everyone irrespective of class, creed, gender, race or wealth must be respected at all times. This is not idle rhetoric; I see this as the only basis on which humanity can build a fair and decent world. Yet here was this man, my equal, probably my superior, kowtowing to me.

So you can understand how I felt. No one had kissed my hand since I was a young doctor in Ireland years before when some elderly patients had done so. And even then, I had felt awkward and embarrassed.

'About how many people live in the district?' I asked, after I had disengaged his hand as politely as I could.

'Many, he replied

'A thousand? ... two thousand? ... une mille ... deux mille?'

'Four thousand ... maybe more....' he replied.

'Count on me. I will have the food here one week from now, I promise' (big man me).

Next day I did the rounds of the International Agencies and friendly embassies in Kigali. This was easy as they were all close to one another. I received a blank everywhere. My last call was to the EU Mission, where I was just too late to see the man in charge. However, I said I'd be back next day and was told that 2.30 p.m. would be a good time.

I did just that. Two thirty came and went while I sat uneasily in the air-conditioned waiting room. I knew that the office closed at three o'clock.

I was now quite on edge. But my luck was in. The man in charge – I cannot remember his name – was just about to leave, but could not do so without passing me. I saw the door to his office open and out he came, beautifully dressed and in an obvious hurry. I blocked his way, politely but firmly. 'Sir' I began 'I wonder if you have a minute to spare.' He was not used to people blocking his way but somehow he sensed that he could not avoid this rather shabbily dressed white man in a tee shirt and shorts. 'Is it urgent? I have an appointment in fifteen minutes in Government buildings.' I took the hint. No time for any preamble.

'I need food to feed 4,000 people and it is urgent. I mean right now if possible. I have tried everywhere and am coming to you in desperation.'

Whether it was my words, my tone or my accent I do not know. But he stopped and looked more closely at me 'Irish? ... You are Irish?' I assured him I was Irish. 'And what part do you come from?' I told him Galway. Did I know Cavan? Not very well I replied. He did not tell me where he came from but I guessed that at least one of his ancestors had hailed from Cavan. For his whole attitude visibly changed and he shook his head in resignation.

He bade me to follow him to an outside office where he introduced me to Simone, a Rwandan, and clearly someone of authority too. 'This man wants us to deliver food to feed for 4000 for say a month, can you organise it Simone?' He then turned to me, shook hands and said Simone would take care of things and then he was gone, possibly to Government Buildings, but more probably to the Club to have a few drinks before dinner.

Simone took details of time and place of delivery and promised that two trucks full of food would arrive the following Tuesday, stipulating that it was up to me to have men there to unload them, and making me promise that I would ensure security and fair distribution. I was delighted, full of my own sense of accomplishment and full of self-importance. I had done it.

Everything went according to plan the next week. The only problem was that the trucks did not arrive until 5 p.m. while I had everyone waiting since before dawn. I was the only white person among the throng waiting for the trucks. I felt uneasy as the hours went by with no sign of them coming. Those around me were getting uneasy too and even restless. By the time the trucks appeared we all heaved a collective sigh of relief and I went home quietly while the food was being distributed.

That night I thanked God for the day past but also asked Him why He did not send the trucks earlier.

And yet the satisfaction one derives from helping a thousand is nothing compared to the satisfaction one gets from helping one person or one family. Large numbers breed anonymity and finally one becomes blasé and begins to treat the whole business of feeding them and supplying their essential needs as just that, a business. There is little or no emotional involvement in such an exercise.

As I watched, three or four dead bodies float down the Rusizi River I felt just as much emotionally involved as if I had seen the thousands of corpses floating in the cavalcade of death, which people reported a month earlier. The Rusizi flows from Lake Kivu to Lake Tanganikya and, when the latter overflows at high tide, to the Congo River. For once, Victoria Nyanza and the Nile miss out.

Children

Children are amazing. Even at the worst of times, they lift and tear your heart simultaneously. You might think they can be bought with a candy bar or a smile but never with money. Wrong. Well almost wrong.

I was on my own with a government official one day discussing the needs of a small rural community situated high up on a hillside. He was a serious man who seldom smiled but who was keen to show me in person the place he hoped I might help.

After visiting the village, we started the descent to the road where government transport awaited us. He kept talking and reeling off the number of houses, per capita income (nil), the coming winter, the lack of schools and the lack of medical facilities and the lack of everything else under the sun as we made our way down through the shrubs and tall grass.

While he was speaking, I became conscious that we were being followed shyly by a group of ragged children who kept their distance but kept going with us all the time.

That day I had a pocket full of one to five dollar bills and after every few paces, I would stick one on a shrub or on a clump of grass without letting my government friend see me. Soon cries and whoops interrupted his list of statistics as the children spotted what I was doing. My companion would look around and shush them away and continue his monologue but I continued to drop notes behind me until he could no longer contain himself.

He turned around and speaking in Kiswahili warned the children to go home or he would personally put them in jail. I nodded sagely in agreement and continued on as if I had done nothing wrong.

He gave me a peculiar look when we got to the road and I wonder if he knew what I had been doing all along. However, he was too polite to mention it on a silent trip back to Kigali.

I tell this unimportant story because I remember everything about it so vividly. I wish you could have been there. I think you would have enjoyed it. I know I did.

Visitation

Sadness comes in all shapes and sizes and I certainly got plenty of it while in Rwanda. However, sadness can sometimes go hand-in-hand with satisfaction and, however fleeting, it is a combination that is delightful for everyone concerned. I was to savour this the day I asked our driver, Jonathon, to bring me to the poorest and the most traumatised homes in Kigali.

We drove the highways and byways of the city and stopped about a dozen times when Jonathon led me on foot to hovels, shacks and makeshift cardboard homes, many of which one approached by narrow pathways that wound in and out and between and behind the more substantial houses.

In almost every home, there would be a few old men and women but few children and fewer young adults. It was hard to see them properly in the dim interiors, just sitting there in the gloom doing nothing. But it was easy to recognise the apathy and hopelessness that pervaded the atmosphere.

Our gifts were meagre. Jonathon would give a bag of sugar or salt or rice and always sweets if there were children. I would slip a ten-dollar bill into the grannies' hand and scribble a note for anyone who was obviously sick to visit the nearest clinic.

Most of all – and this is without a doubt – our visits brought a fleeting moment of happiness and hope to these families. There was much hugging and many tears and always a genuine 'thank you for not abandoning us' written on every face.

I cannot say this without sounding maudlin but truly, the greatest gift one can bring is one's own presence, there in the flesh, sharing the grief, the hurt and the sorrow of those who feel abandoned.

To know that you are not forgotten is a priceless gift.

One of the jobs we had was to refurnish and repair the school at Rwesero. The school lay on the banks of Lake Muhazi, a long thin lake that runs east–west, not far from Kigali. Even a very talented writer, much less myself, could not portray accurately what I saw on my first visit. Two months earlier 10,000 Tutsi had been murdered – mostly hacked to death – there, and the smell of death still hung in the air. The walls of the classrooms were streaked with dried blood. Pools of congealed blood were still on floors, which were blanketed even now with buzzing insatiable insects. Desks were smashed, copybooks torn and scattered about, and every fixture was ripped out and carried away. The usual children's drawings, that had decorated the rooms in better times, were smeared with blood, and the pictures of Mickey Mouse, Dumbo the elephant and other cartoon characters stared pathetically and accusingly at us.

All the bodies had been removed when the remnants of a fearful local population had come back from hiding, but somehow the abandoned classrooms told their own story more graphically and more suggestively now that they were silent and empty.

Things are so different now. It is hard to believe that anything bad ever happened there. Today you can stay in any of a number of lovely hotels on the shores of Lake Muhazi. Swimming, bird watching, hiking, fishing and exploring the lush tropical countryside, so rich in exotic flora and fauna, are very popular with tourists. Rwesero is now a very safe and friendly place, where the shadows of the past seem, on the surface at least, to have been dissipated by the courage and hope of the local people.

Gradually, over the second half of 1994, things settled down and a kind of normality returned to everyday life in Rwanda. Not so for the two million Hutus who were now on the run. Soon the world began to hear of their plight as they streamed over the borders into neighbouring countries and were housed in makeshift camps. One of these camps was near the town of Goma in the DCR. Goma became the site of horrific slaughter as rival Hutu factions, including the Congolese army, sought to annihilate one another.

I spent Christmas of 1995 in Giseyni, a small town just across the border from Goma, which was within walking distance. My travelling companion was Deirdre Ruane, a young red-headed Irish nurse, who has since dedicated her life to working for impoverished African communities. Deirdre and I worked well together and two of us made a very effective team doing lots of things not strictly medical. This included organising local groups to set up small commercial operations, overseeing the rebuilding of damaged houses, initiating the construction of simple 'boma' homes for the dispossessed and buying provisions such as food, furniture, mattresses, seeds and farming utensils and distributing these where we felt they were most needed.

Our Christmas break in Giseyni, on the shores of Lake Kivu, was indeed idyllic, even if our Christmas dinner in the local Concern house was forgettable. That afternoon I walked to Goma with a Spanish teacher who had worked there for many years. He advised me not to go into the camp and for once, I was smart and took his advice. Heroes are for novels.

Annette

It was our policy to employ Rwandans whenever possible. In this way, we liaised more effectively with locals, sourced materials at better prices, identified those with genuine needs and, of course, all salaries fed into the local economy.

Annette Mugwaneza was only sixteen years of age when she joined our team. We came across Annette wandering, apparently aimlessly, on the roadside outside Kigali. She really had nowhere to go. Her family had been almost completely wiped out during the genocide and her home had been ransacked and set on fire. After her primary schooling in Kigali, she had been sent to boarding school in Uganda where she became an articulate and accomplished young lady. Despite her terrible ordeals, she was still able to smile timidly at us and, on a sudden but good impulse, we asked her to join our team.

She spoke excellent English and immediately agreed to work in whatever capacity she might be most useful. Initially she did small jobs around the house that we had rented, but soon it was clear that Annette had abilities way beyond her sixteen years of age. She quickly began to help with managing things for us. Her knowledge of local people and local politics was invaluable and we began to rely on her advice when making decisions on who to help, what people to see and how to get things done.

Her organisational skills became clear when she stood in for anyone who was on leave or absent because of sickness and her loyalty was proved by the many warnings she gave us when otherwise we might have been taken in by smooth talking locals, who were charging exorbitant prices for their services. Annette was a lovely person, easy to work with, obliging, trustworthy and kind to all.

This kindness extended particularly to the mothers and children that we worked with and it is little wonder that, when we left Rwanda, Annette was put in complete charge of our operations there. Afterwards she started a new organisation called 'Trust and Care' to help children orphaned during the genocide. I quote from the *Independent Newspaper* (UK) of August 2015:

'There are an estimated 300,000 children in Rwanda – children whose parents perished in the 1994 massacres or in the chaos that followed. ..... Nine out of 10 children saw corpses and body parts piled high, a third witnessed rapes and other violent assaults, three out of five were threatened with death and nine out of 10 thought they were going to die....'

These are the children that Annette, now married and a mother herself, was trying to help.

I have few personal reminders of my days in Rwanda. One of the few that I have is a photograph of Annette and her family which came to me by a circuitous route a few years ago. There she is with her children and, standing as large as life with her, is Dominic, her eldest son. So my name – if not my work – remains on in the new generation of Rwandans who will someday forget the blackest 100 days their country has ever seen.

Kofi Annan

It would be a mistake to think that life for Aid workers is all doom and gloom. Even in the worst of times, volunteers from different NGOs meet together and have a 'party'.

I first met Kofi Annan at such a party in Kigali where, like myself, I think he was only waiting for a chance to escape. We found mutual kinship in our conversation (near the door) and, although I did not realise this soft-spoken Ghanaian was destined for a high office, it came as no surprise to me when he did. Within a year, he was appointed by Boutros-Ghali as his Special Representative in the former Yugoslavia, and two years later, in 1997, replaced him as Secretary General of the United Nations.

I imagine that, as a career diplomat, his hands were largely tied and he could not railroad a policy through the labyrinth of intrigue, political posturing and self-interest that bedevils all large international institutions. But I am certain he tried his best.

Kofi and I left together that night, perhaps I should say escaped together, and went our different ways. I remember it was a dark though starlight night and, as we said goodbye, I felt I had met a true gentleman.

I never met him personally again and I am certain that he does not even remember meeting me.

Soft Hearts in Tough Men

I must add a small story to my experiences in Rwanda. This time it is a good news story.

Mother Teresa's nuns, the Missionary Sisters of Charity, had a home for the dying in Kigali which I visited regularly, to bring whatever I could beg, borrow or steal.

Sometimes I would have nothing to bring apart from twenty US dollars. I knew the Sisters could buy quite a lot with twenty dollars but I also knew that I was welcome when I brought nothing. Many of the Sisters were Asian but the majority were African. During the genocide, they had hidden people from the marauding mobs and so, unlike some other convents, were held in high esteem by the new regime.

I found that all the Sisters in the home for the dying were patient and kind to those in their care irrespective or class, creed, colour or gender and it was my privilege to see them at work as they tended the dying or fed those incapable of feeding themselves.

They did work of which I am incapable. For it is easy to spend ten minutes doing it, but consider spending a whole day, a whole week, *all your life* as they do, and then you will begin to appreciate the kind of people they are.

Men and women were accommodated in four long low buildings, about twenty in each, making a full complement of eighty for ten sisters to mind. Since deaths were a daily occurrence, there was a quick turnover, and yet there were people squatting on the road outside, hoping to get their loved ones into the Sister's care.

I commented to the Sisters on how dark the low ceilinged 'wards' were, but of course there was no electricity and Tilley lamps would be dangerous. This meant darkness from 6 p.m. to 6 a.m. each day and clearly this posed a big problem for the Sisters and their cares alike.

It happened that a group of British soldiers was stationed nearby and I mentioned this to one of them. He was a big tough guy with a very pronounced British accent – meaning we hardly understood each other. Yet he got the drift of my dilemma and immediately said he would do something about it.

Within a week, a few ordinary army privates – there were no officers involved – drove up to the Sisters compound and unloaded and then installed a beautiful new generator. They also delivered enough gas to keep it going for a month with a promise to resupply gas for the foreseeable future. All this was done without charge and done with lots of laughter and smart badinage.

I asked whether they had got permission to give away the generator. I gathered by innuendo that they had nicked it from their stores. I don't think that was true, I think they wanted to shock me, but yet I am not really certain that they bothered to seek official permission, which would likely have taken several months 'going through channels' before final approval.

Thank you England.

A Pathetic Footnote

This concerns Laurencie, the nurse attendant I mentioned earlier, who first helped us in Kyanza Health Centre. I have just come across a letter from her dated 25 January 1995. It goes thus:

Dr Dominique

First I greet you so much. We have received your news but you don't know ours. To-day our news is too bad. My husband Ndenzi Meloine is dead, assassinated on 21st January this year, so I am not well today because I have five orphans....
God Bless you

Yours
Mukoimurenti Laurencie

My reply is rather bland but then I had many letters like this one to reply to. It went:

Dear Laurencie... Thank you for remembering me. I hope your new baby is well and that the family is managing things alright. Times will improve slowly and I am sure the rest of 1995 will turn out better for you and your family. Keep on trying. I too remember Ndenzi with much love and sadness but I know you have had such a hard time that nothing I can say will ever ease you.

God bless you and your family
Dr Dom

On 10th February, Anne Malone, who had stayed in Rwanda, wrote to me concerning the details of Ndenzi's murder. It was a long letter and I only give a small part of it here:

Dear Dom,

It is with great sorrow that I write to tell you of the events leading up to Ndenzi's death. Augustin, the night guard, was responsible for looting both the Health Centre and Eugene's house after the April massacres (Eugene was the caretaker).

Anne went on to explain that both Ndenzi and Eugene reported Augustin to the authorities and that in reprisal, Augustin and five of his friends waylaid Ndenzi on 21 January 1995 and battered him to death. They lowered his body into a deep well.

But it was discovered, and Augustin and his five accomplices were thrown into Kigali Central Prison and later convicted.

Anne's letter finished with an account of how the work of Refugee Trust was progressing and how happy she was that we were the third NGO to be officially accepted by the new Government just being pipped by Médecins sans Frontières and World Vision. Not bad out of one hundred and fifty nine NGOs that had applied for recognition and of which the majority were rejected.

I made several visits to Rwanda over the next few years and each time found that life was steadily getting back to some kind of normality.

I do not know what the future holds for that land. The unspeakable hurt of the genocide is fading but people's memories will never fade.

Official figures issued by the Rwandan Government put the death toll at between one and two million of which 10 per cent were Hutu. A conservative estimate by the UN suggests that 800,000 were slaughtered in the first 100 days that is 8,000 a day, 333 an hour and 5–6 a minute.

One of the iconic tangible reminders for all generations to come is to be found in Nyamata, 30 km south of Kigali. Thousands of people fled to the Catholic Church there seeking sanctuary. But instead of sanctuary they were brutally raped, tortured, butchered and burnt alive in one of the most savage episodes of the genocide. It is estimated that 50,000 Tutsis were murdered there. The torn blood stained clothing of thousands of those massacred is draped across the pews along with piles of skulls, one of which is still impaled with a spear.

Nyamata church is as much a genocide memorial as the Holocaust museum in Jerusalem or the Nazi camp at Auschwitz.

CHAPTER 15

THE BALKANS BURN

Medjugorge

My wife and I first visited Medjugorge in 1986 as pilgrims. At that time it was a quiet backwater, a place history seemed to have passed by, in which people lived lives just as their grandparents did and in which the possibility of it becoming a place of major international pilgrimage seemed absurd. Our visit was peaceful and although we were conscious of local political unease, the idea of a major war never entered our heads until we met Donna McGettigan. Donna, the 'girl from Donegal' was to become one of the most important contacts between Ireland and Medjugorje in the subsequent war. Originally, she had been a guide with Joe Walsh Tours, but she fell in love with Medjugorje and decided to stay there permanently. After a short time, she opened a hostel in the centre of the town and, as far as I could see, also managed 'Paddy Tours' single handed. Donna, now Donna McGettigan-Ostojic, still lives there.

She has written several books about the apparitions in Medjugorje and I can vouch personally that she not only believes them but is also a level-headed Donegal woman whose word should not be lightly put aside. She is also a hospitable and generous person who might have exploited her position to make a fortune from tourists and pilgrims, but never did so.

Medjugorje in War Time

It was on foot of Donna's reports of killings and plundering in and around Medjugorje by the Chetniks and by their sworn enemies the Ustaše that Liam Prendergast and I decided to visit Medjugorje in 1992 and see the situation for ourselves. We were good travelling companions and never got on each other's nerves despite being together day and night for two weeks. At least Liam never got on my nerves. And I hope I did not get on his either.

We flew first to a small airport in Austria where we spent the night in a nearby hotel. Liam had been a general in the Irish army and was a meticulous person in every way. He was also an extremely religious man and every night, before getting into bed, he would kneel down and say the rosary. He put all his feeling into the prayers and I knew he was genuine. I joined him in prayer and wondered what we were getting ourselves into. I was not familiar with the situation in the Balkans at that time and in truth my thoughts were more on South Sudan where I was due to go shortly afterwards.

To look at Liam you would not have thought him an army man. He was slim, hardy and a little below average height. He certainly did not fit the popular picture of an army general such as Patton, Eisenhower, Rommel, Zhukov or De Gaulle – I except little Monty!

Liam was not a trivial person. He was a serious intense individual and truly committed to his duty, whatever it was and wherever it would lead. He had a phenomenal memory for names, places and dates, and this was in complete contrast to me, whose life is a constant struggle with trying to put names on faces, faces on names and dates on events.

If Liam was somewhat pedantic and predictable, then these traits were more than offset by his dedication, sincerity and loyalty and a nature that was generous to a fault. He was indeed a man of integrity – a rare breed indeed.

Since the airport at Mostar was now closed to civilian traffic, it meant we would have to fly to Split, in Croatia. Mostar is only a twenty minutes' run from Medjugorje but it would take us up to three hours to get there from Split. That did not bother us as long as we arrived safely in Split, which we eventually did in a small plane operated by a small airline.

On later visits, I discovered the beauties of Split, one of the oldest towns on the Dalmatian coast. The Palace of Diocletian is very well preserved and is a focal point for the tourist, but this it is just one of many buildings and sites which bear testament to a succession of rulers and invaders over the past centuries.

Split airport was uncannily quiet when we landed in our small aeroplane. We were the only arrival and there was just one other plane on the tarmac. Several HVO (Croatian) soldiers eyed us as we disembarked but none of them bothered to halt us or ask us our business. Customs waved us through in a perfunctory manner and we were outside the airport in less than fifteen minutes. There a young man in an old black Mercedes met us. He was parked on the double yellow lines outside the exit door but was chatting to a HVO soldier which obviously circumvented normal parking rules. The moment he saw Liam his face lit up and he hurried to help with our cases after embracing Liam warmly. Liam, a regular visitor to Medjugorje, obviously knew him well and I was certainly pleased that he did. We had carried parcels of medicine, canned food, powdered milk and children's toys from Ireland, but they seemed pathetically small in the voluminous boot of the old Mercedes.

I sat in the back, glad to avoid trying to make conversation with the driver. In any case, he only spoke to Liam who kept plying him with questions about the 'war' and life in general in Medjugorje. Our journey passed quickly and we saw no sign of the terrible things that were being reported. However, there was little traffic and far fewer people on the road than might have been expected.

We spent a week in Medjugorje but it was long enough to give away all we had and begin to understand the plight of the people. We ate in Donna's one night and she told us tales of killings and abductions that were hard to believe. I determined privately to go back again before things got out of hand completely. Next time I would only bring those medical supplies that I could see were urgently needed such as morphine, antibiotics, dressings, needles, syringes and simple surgical sets.

Liam continued to kneel and say the Rosary every night no matter how many he had said during the day. Once again, I joined him, meaning it more than on the first night in Austria.

A Private Visit

People at home were profoundly moved by events in the Balkans, especially by events around Medjugorje which was a place so dear to many Irish hearts. As a result, they held table quizzes, coffee mornings, fashion shows and ran raffles and church gate collections to raise money for those suffering in the Balkans. I know that I received cash, cheques and donations of medicines which the donors expected me to deliver *personally and in full*. So with this responsibility in mind, I set off alone to do just that.

Even a few weeks had made a profound difference. The land was now burning and no one was safe. I entered the Balkans again through Austria and made my way to Trogir, where I was to spend the first night in the home of a Croatian friend of Liams.

Trogir is a truly beautiful historic walled town that lies about 20 km west of Split but is much closer to the airport. The old town is situated on a small island in the Adriatic linked by bridges to the much larger island of Čiovo and the mainland. Thankfully, Trogir was untouched by the war for it is a real gem. Liam's friend lived on the island in a house that must have been hundreds of years old. He was an ebullient person, warm and welcoming and absolutely delighted to have someone listen to his opinions about Tubman, the war and the world. I spent a very happy night with him but we were both a little tipsy by the time we went to bed.

The following afternoon I left for Medjugorje. My host provided a rather dilapidated car and a rather dilapidated grim-faced driver. But I was content that he would take me safely to my destination.

Once past Split, we slowed down and entered a series of byroads. This was to avoid army checkpoints and brigands. In so doing, I began to appreciate that this was not just a paper war, but was a real one, in which danger was as real as the road in front of us.

As the minutes turned to hours, my grim-faced driver became more and more uneasy. Finally, we passed a certain fork in the road after which he relaxed and announced that we were now safe, and would be in Medjugorje in half an hour. He actually smiled at this stage. However, it was almost dusk when we rolled into the town. It appeared completely deserted and even the silent houses looked threatening against the darkening sky. We stopped outside a non-descript building but before the driver got out he told me to stay where I was until he called me. He then disappeared around the back of the building and I was left sitting in the car looking after him anxiously, for this was not the kind of reception I was expecting.

After a few moments, he returned, put a finger to his lips and beckoned me to follow him. I got out of the car and closed the door quietly then I followed him around the side of the house, passing several shuttered windows on the way. This added to the eerie atmosphere. He stopped at the back door and knocked lightly. The door opened almost instantly and a young woman stood aside to let us pass. She smiled and motioned us both to come inside. We entered a large room heated by a log stove that hissed and crackled loudly as the buzz of conversation from those within suddenly stopped.

Several men were sitting around a central table drinking coffee and all arose as we entered. A grizzly faced elderly man with strong Slavic features stepped forward. He beamed at me and gave me a bear hug. 'Ah…it is good to see any friend of Liams …come sit down, we have been expecting you …Demir will take your things inside.' I was then the recipient of another hug. I felt a grizzly stubble rub my cheek and a hot vodka-laden breath added to my discomfort. But I smiled to everyone and sat down gratefully on the chair the woman pushed over to me. I hoped to avoid having any more hugs. But I got up again to shake hands with everyone in the room as they filed over to me one by one. No more hugs!

At last, with more scraping of chairs, we all sat down and the woman brought out a big pot of well-brewed coffee. It tasted good. She then produced two bottles of vodka (well, a clear fluid in a bottle) and planted a tray full of small glasses on the table so that everyone could help himself. Only the grizzly man seemed to speak English. He now addressed Demir.

'Thank God you made it…things are getting worse. What was your journey like from Trogir? … Demir … Did you get kerosene? Did you hear such and such a village was attacked? … what were the roads like?' Villages here have unpronounce-able names.

Demir just nodded, probably unable to take in so many questions in English at the same time. But without waiting for a reply, the grizzly man turned to me once more saying how delighted he was to see me and how much they appreciated help of any sort from their Irish friends and so on, until his English faltered. I wondered privately if he would say the same things no matter where I came from. Or am I cynic? Lots was then said in the local language so I missed most of the conversation, but I knew I was welcome, and this was reinforced by the fine meal that followed, all served by the same woman who had let us in. There was chicken, salad, fruit and corn plus good local red wine. And of course more vodka.

I need not say more about this trip. I gave money and gift parcels to the locals and Fr Slavko put the medical supplies in his room near the church. He thanked me by letting me be present in the room when the visionaries were having an apparition. There were about five of us there, all privileged people. It was a moving experience.

Slavko Barbarić was a Fransiscan priest who promoted Medjugorje tirelessly and was intimately involved with the visionaries and with the pilgrims.

He died at 3.30 p.m. on Friday 24 November 2000 immediately after doing the Way of the Cross on Krizevac Hill. I always found him to be a holy man who worked ceaselessly for others. However, some found his call to austerity too severe and his manner cold.

In the days that followed, I took part in the general life of the village including prayer in St James Church and climbing barefoot to the Holy Cross on Mt Krizevac. I promised myself that I would collect more money at home as soon as I could. It would be used to rebuild houses, buy food and medicine and provide the dispossessed with a means of living or even of escape to the West. There was always some way to get money to Medjugorje, always couriers willing to cross over the mountains from Austria and always someone willing to take the risk.

Needless to say, I got back to Dublin safe and sound and much chastened but, more than ever, I was determined to go back again if the opportunity arose. That would not happen for another three years.

Sarajevo

Sarajevo, the capital of Bosnia and Herzegovina, nestles in the valley of the Miljacka River and sits in a deep saucer, surrounded by high hills on almost every side. The old historic city lies on the northeastern bank of the river while to the west and south there is a sprawl of ugly apartment blocks and industrial estates which clearly follow the pattern of the dismal architecture of the communist era.

The three great monotheistic Faiths have coexisted in harmony for many centuries in Sarajevo and you will find the Roman Catholic and Eastern Orthodox cathedrals almost juxtaposed to the Emperors Mosque. The Sarajevo Synagogue – the only functioning Synagogue in Sarajevo today – is but a stone thrown across the river.

All these places of worship are in the 'old city', the heart of Sarajevo, the place where for centuries people of all faiths and none have met, drank coffee, played chess and talked endlessly as friends do.

The Start of the Siege

It is said that the spark that set off the siege was an attack by a Muslim mob on a Serb wedding in downtown Sarajevo on

1 March 1992 – barely a month before my trip to Bosnia with Liam Prendergast. During the attack, the groom's father was killed and many of the guests were seriously injured.

Serb paramilitaries responded by setting up barricades, by blocking the entrance to government buildings and by placing snipers in apartment buildings. These snipers shot and killed people indiscriminately and were to become a dreaded and hated feature of the succeeding siege. However, within hours, the Serbs were confronted by thousands of ordinary Sarajevo citizens and the city began to function again. Things now moved fast.

In two short days, on 3rd March, the Government in Sarajevo proclaimed the Independent Republic of Bosnia and Herzegovina. Within months, the EU recognised the new state and its secession from Yugoslavia became a *fait accompli*. This was a signal for widespread fighting throughout the country between Serbs and the predominantly Muslim Government forces. The Bosnian War had begun.

In the months that followed, Sarajevo was thrown into turmoil in which those living in different parts of the city, and even in adjacent apartment blocks, took up arms against one another. Signs of *Pagite Snajper* (Beware Sniper!) or *Pazi-Snajper* (Watch out-Sniper!) appeared everywhere. And, as if the internal fighting was not enough, the city soon became surrounded by the Yugoslav People's Army. The encirclement was complete by 5th April. The siege of Sarajevo had officially begun.

Only those who lived through the siege can describe the next four years. My experiences pale in comparison with theirs and it would be presumptuous and wrong of me to suggest otherwise. However, I was there towards the end when the weary city had virtually lost all hope.

The Siege

The siege of Sarajevo was the longest urban siege in modern history. The siege proper started on 5 April 1992, and lasted until 29 February 1996, a total of 1425 days. The besieged were the citizens of Sarajevo and the Bosniak army; the besiegers were first the Yugoslav Army and then the Army of Republika Srpska. In most people eyes, it was Bosniak versus Serb, and Muslim versus Christian. But this oversimplifies matters. Many Muslim Bosniaks served in the attacking army and many Orthodox Serbs fought to repel them.

At least 14,000 people were killed in Sarajevo itself. These deaths were due to sniper fire, indiscriminate mortar attacks and relentless shelling from tanks and gun emplacements on the surrounding hills.

Probably a greater number died from a lack of medical attention, a lack of drugs, undernutrition and infectious diseases – especially those carried by polluted water. Old people suffered from the cruel cold of successive Sarajevo winters and pregnant mothers often gave birth to their babies in appalling conditions.

The Bosnian army defending the city – with amazing foresight – started to build a tunnel as early as March 1992. The tunnel was constructed so that it linked the besieged city with Bosnian held territory on the other side of the Serb lines. You entered it through an ordinary looking house in the Bosnian controlled suburb of Butmir and emerged in a similarly innocuous looking way at Dobrinja, having passed beneath the airport, which the UN controlled from early on.

All kinds of merchandise passed through the tunnel. Much of it was food; but it was also a conduit for arms for the beleaguered defenders. People slipped through both ways and many of the escapees told of the daily atrocities that were being perpetrated inside the city where groups of paramilitaries on both sides often fought one another from adjacent buildings.

Journey to Hell

This was probably the strangest journey I ever made. It was certainly the most dangerous one and, in many ways, was a foolhardy undertaking.

We had all been watching the terrible events in the Balkans with increasing distress and increasing anger, as night after night our TV screens showed live pictures of people being killed in cold blood and of streams of refugees haggard and distraught struggling along war-strafed roads. We saw cities, towns and villages that had been reduced to amorphous masses of rubble. And we saw cities in which the only sign of life was the appearance of a mangy dog or furtive cat scavenging amid the debris for whatever they could find to eat.

Little things, like a child's doll or a twisted bicycle lying on the road, reminded us that not long ago families lived normal lives, did normal things and worked and played and ate and drank, just like us.

The destruction of Vukovar and the bombing of Sulie-man Bridge in Mostar were just two of the mindless ravages of historic sites that shocked the civilised world. But above all, it was the helpless plight of the people of Sarajevo, caught up in a slaughter, unprecedented since the WWII, that moved many of us in the West, to get up, go out and help – not just with words and monetary donations – but by actively sharing in the suffering of the people and by actively putting whatever skill we might have at their service.

I felt I could do something. I was a medical doctor with a lot of experience in crisis situations and I would also raise money to give directly to as many people as possible. There was nothing heroic in this decision. I felt I had to make it and act on it. In this, I had the full backing of Doreen and the children, and it is to them that any credit is due.

It was not difficult to organise my trip. I was the only doctor on the board of Refugee Trust and we had already a small office in Sarajevo. So I was the obvious one to send out and all the board members accepted my offer readily. Tom O'Grady, a feisty Brother of the Order of St John of God, administered our office in Sarajevo so I would be going to a fellow Irishman in a ready-made setup.

We kept in touch with Tom via satellite phone because the siege of Sarajevo blocked ordinary phone calls, and although one could theoretically enter or exit via the 'airport tunnel', the Bosniaks kept a strict control of all movement through it and I doubt that they would let me use it. On the other hand, there was no way that I could have been granted safe passage through the Serb lines. I would have to be smuggled in.

I took a suitcase and a cheap duffle bag – a backpack, no more. The latter contained a few personal things and the case was crammed with medical items such as suture sets, antibiotics, morphine, pethidine (demerol) and codeine tablets. I carried my passport and a few dollars in a zipped pocket inside my jacket and wore a canvas money belt containing up to 30,000 d-marks around my body. I shudder to think how naïve I was. I was a fair game for anyone on any side in a conflict about which, at that time, I knew practically nothing except that it was bloody, vicious and wrong.

As my plane lifted off from Dublin Airport I wondered what was in store.

The Adriatic looked particularly lovely as we crossed from Italy towards the Dalmatian coast. I think there are few coastlines in the world to rival that which extends from Trieste in the north to the Ionian Sea in the south. But I was thinking of other things as we finally descended and landed gently in a military airport outside Split, half way down the coast of Croatia

First, I had to wait outside the plane for my luggage to be thrown out and that took some time. Then I had to go through immigration in the terminal itself. I must have looked like a harmless lumbering peasant, as with one hand I lugged a rather tattered brown suitcase while at the same time, with my other hand, I dragged my duffel bag behind me. One of the straps of the duffel bag had snapped in two when I was pulling it down from the overhead locker in the plane, and this small thing caused me much irritation, for now I only had my mouth free to transport my passport. I clasped this precious document firmly between clenched teeth and approached the immigration desk. A tired looking middle-aged fellow in a rather grubby uniform sat on a kitchen chair behind a small brown wooden desk. He looked kindly at me. A proper terrorist would not have come in such a bedraggled way. He would have swaggered up, calm and confident. Instead here was I, hot and flustered and presenting him with a saliva soaked passport.

After a moment of hesitation, he waved me through with something approaching a grin on his face. I breathed a sigh of relief. It is always a little tense passing through immigration in foreign countries.

There were neither 'Welcome to Croatia' signs anywhere nor any other indication that I was welcome. Yet I was relieved. I have spent many hours in many countries waiting in queues, often the wrong queue. Here there was no queue. Presumably sane people wanted to get out of the Balkans, not get in.

I was hoping that Tom might be there to meet me but there was no sign of him. However, I was not too worried. I knew that someone would turn up. I have no idea why I was so confident, for Tom's plans could easily have gone astray. But no, I was hardly waiting ten minutes, when a tall dark young man approached me.

'You Doktor Dom, Irish?' he asked in a thick Slavic accent, which I would get used to over the next few weeks. I told him I was and that I was happy to see him. He obligingly lifted my heavy suitcase and beckoned me to follow him. We made our way outside to a very dusty and very old black sedan of indeterminate age and indeterminate make. But it had a large boot, which easily accommodated my entire luggage. I sank down gratefully into the passenger seat, which sagged deeply beneath my weight. Perhaps it had carried much heavier people than me in previous times or perhaps it was used to carry heavy milk churns or sacks of vegetables.

'We go safe house. Brother Tomas leave yesterday. He say he sorry not able wait any longer. He meet you Sarajevo.' This all sounded fine. Obviously Tom knew I was coming and had arranged things for me. I sat back more relaxed now than before. I was on my way.

My driver, whose name I cannot remember except that it ended in -ic (pronounced 'itch') was a man of few words. In my mind, I christened him 'Itch'. At least that was easy to remember.

It was clearly an effort for him to speak English but he did manage to assure me the Tom was safe, that he was taking the mountain route (whatever that was) and that Itch's brother was escorting him to Sarajevo, which he possibly entered via the tunnel. At least that is what I understood from him. I still do not know if Itch was a Bosnian or a Croat or a Serb. In time, I began to recognise typical examples of these people but initially I confess that I often confused one with the other. 'And how will I get to Sarajevo?' There was no immediate answer. We then lapsed into silence.

Eventually we turned into a laneway that led to a small farmhouse somewhere on the outskirts of Split, from which we could see the sparkling Adriatic lapping the shore. 'We see' he remarked as we pulled up to a stop outside the red painted door of a farmhouse. 'We see *what*' I wondered.

I followed him inside and discovered the house was empty but that a meal for two had been left on the kitchen table. We both ate in silence and once we were finished he showed me a bedroom and indicated that he would be back for me in the morning. Then he left. I was glad to be alone but doubts crept into my mind as to what exactly I was doing here.

Early next day he drove me down into the city and put me on a bus heading in the general direction of Zenica where I 'should meet a contact. He take you from there.' My contact was a 'catholic priest' who lived in St Elijah's church. That was it. The word vague hardly describes these instructions.

Main roads were deemed unsafe and we would travel on byroads to Zenica as far as possible. It would be an arduous four hours' journey, but Itch assured me it was the safest route for me to travel. I had the comfort of having plenty of German Marks – in addition to US dollars – and both currencies were gratefully accepted everywhere. No doubt they would later be exchanged on the black market for food and clothes or else hoarded carefully for future use, perhaps even as a means of escaping to the West. So I paid the driver in deutschmarks and found a window seat somewhere to the rear of the bus.

The bus set off from an esplanade near the sea and, at that early hour, the Adriatic looked sour and forbidding, no longer the deep blue of the previous day. My few fellow travellers looked sour and forbidding too. They spoke little and smoked incessantly. Almost all were men. No one sat beside me. It would have been difficult anyway. I had my suitcase and duffel bag squarely on the seat and, since I kept resolutely looking out the window, I avoided eye contact with any busy-body who might have liked to share my company. This is a ploy commonly used by those travelling on buses and trains when they do not want to share a seat with anyone. It usually works too.

After running south for some miles along the seaboard, we took a left fork and started to go due east. The road began to deteriorate and the bus continually spluttered and stalled as we climbed hill after hill penetrating deeper and deeper into the heart of the land. There was no discernible border crossing between Croatia and Bosnia and by now, I was one of only three passengers left on the bus. After another fifteen minutes, I was the sole occupant and my uneasiness at being alone turned into a definite feeling of worry when the bus finally stalled and stopped in the middle of nowhere – as far as I could see. The driver got out of his seat and shrugged despairingly at me as if to say there was nothing I could do now but wait or walk.

It seemed he favoured the latter because he kept pointing along the road saying 'Zenica … Zenica…' and then he turned to me and in clear body language indicated that I should get out and walk. 'Finish ... finish…' he intoned with a finality that left me in no doubt that the bus was to blame not him. 'Bus no go ... No go.'

I kept saying 'How far? ... How far Zenica? … Is a long way, No?' My pidgin English seemed appropriate at this point. No point in using extra words when he probably did not under-stand anything I was saying. Again, he shrugged his shoulders and, as if inspired, grinned and said 'No problem…No prob-lem.' Undoubtedly, he had picked this up from some American TV show and it sounded good to him.

I could do nothing but get out of the bus, gather my belong-ings and trample in the general direction of Zenica. We waved good-bye to each other and so I left him there, standing beside the bus, a forlorn figure if I ever saw one. However, I happened to glance back as I reached the top of the next hill and the bus was no longer there. Either the driver wanted to get rid of me or the engine had miraculously revived itself. I suspect there was no miracle.

It was now afternoon and I was both hungry and thirsty. I was also angry with the driver but resigned to my fate. The sun was well up in the sky yet dark clouds scudded across its face making me wonder if even the weather was turning against me.

I reckoned I would walk to the nearest house, buy some food and water and perhaps bed down for the night. But I was luckier than that. I had been only twenty minutes or so walking when I heard the unmistakable sound of a vehicle cresting the hill behind me. Unfortunately, it was not a bus, much less 'my' bus, but an old weary looking truck with a florid-faced driver all alone in the cab. Good fortune smiled on me again. I stood in the centre of the road, better call it a path, and blocked his way while waving my hands in a frantic move to make him stop – before he should run into me.

In those days, stopping for a stranger was a risky business. I might have been anyone. I might easily have robbed him, hurt him, taken his truck or even murdered him. But fortune was on my side once more. He pulled up within a few feet of me and leaned out the window while he said something – probably quite rude – about people wanting to be killed by standing in the middle of the road. I gestured that I wanted a lift while at the same time climbing up on the passenger side and letting myself in beside him.

I said 'Zen-*icha*' in my best Croatian accent, emphasising the '*icha*' part at the end. He nodded, smiled and got the truck going again, hardly noticing me. I was very relieved.

I remember little of the road but do recall seeing a beautiful monastery on the side of a lake, which I later learned was the Franciscan monastery of Tomislavgrad or Duvno as it is often called. The monastery, like so many others in the East, is dedicated to the brothers, Cyril and Methodius, the Apostles of the Slavs, and now co-patrons of Europe. I understand it was called after the emperor Tomislav on the occasion of his coronation in 924 AD. I remember thinking what a lovely location and hoped I might visit it sometime again.

All the time, the driver and I managed a very happy conversation together, despite not understanding much of what either was saying. In my relief, I produced a half litre bottle of *Paddy* – Irish whiskey – which we both shared liberally and I believe this broke down barriers more than anything else. I often buy a few half-litre plastic bottles of whiskey when travelling abroad. One never knows how useful they can be. Certainly, it made the journey pass happily for both of us and, by the time he eventually deposited me at St Elijahs, we were both very happy men.

Deposited is the correct word because I literally fell out of the truck when I opened the door. I had forgotten how high up I was, and on taking a step down found that there was no ground beneath my foot. So I landed ignominiously on my backside much to the amusement of my red-faced friend and to the astonishment of a little boy who happened to be watching us. I was angry with myself and mortified, and got up instantly as if I were made of rubber, although my body ached all over, especially my nether regions. 'I'm fine' I said to no one in particular and grinned falsely, dusting myself down as if I had fallen on a soft mattress instead of on hard concrete. The truck driver grinned and with a wave of his hand and a toot of his horn, he vanished from my life forever.

We are merely ships in the night passing one another down the years, forgetting names, places, faces, things we did together, debts we owe, making promises we will never keep and have no real intention of keeping. *C'est la vie*. I was now alone. And yet, in a real sense, I was beginning to understand Cicero when he remarked that you are 'never less alone than when alone'. I never understood that quote when I was a child.

The courtyard on which I was so ingloriously deposited lay to the left-hand side of the main church as seen from the road. Having picked myself up, I crossed towards the side of the church where a short flight of grey stone steps led to an iron-studded door, clearly the entrance to the priests' quarters. After a few hefty thumps and a wait that seemed interminable, another door opened to my right-hand side. I should have noticed this other door for there was a sign pointing to it on the door that I was banging.

A middle-aged woman was framed in the opening and looked at me quizzically. The striking feature about her was her hair, which was ginger coloured, a rarity in those parts. Otherwise, she looked no different from any other middle-aged woman in Bosnia. She was short in stature with a shapeless figure and she had the face of a woman far beyond her years. Her face was lined and prematurely aged and her spade-like hands bespoke years of drudgery and hard work. Nonetheless, when I introduced myself 'Dokita ... Irelandaise...want priest who speak English ... Anglais...' she understood immediately, and she beamed at me with a warm motherly smile. She beckoned me forward taking my suitcase from me and asked me to wait in the hallway until she fetched a priest. Somehow, I felt at ease here and at least I would have a place to lie down for the night. So I waited patiently wondering what would happen next.

When the English-speaking priest arrived, I was surprised that he was so young. To my shame, I cannot remember his name but I think he was a Dominican Friar or at least had kinship with the Dominicans. He certainly was delighted to hear that my first name was Dominic.

I followed him along the hallway and up a wide stairway, the far end of which led to a landing off which there were several rooms. He then opened a door immediately to our left, which turned out to be an office of sorts. A large table covered with papers and files dominated it. There was a book-lined wall on one side with shelving that went almost to the ceiling. Tapestries with biblical scenes covered the opposite wall, while facing the door was a large bay window overlooking a small courtyard.

My host's English was excellent but I had the impression that I was not a particularly wanted guest when, with a shrug of his shoulders, he told me that I would have to sleep on the floor between the desk and window. 'We have no spare rooms' he explained and on retrospect I can quite understand his distant attitude. He had never met me before, I was a foreigner, I could be an informer and I could be spying on the church. And why on earth would anyone want to go to Sarajevo in the first place?

But Brother Tom's name was enough for him to take me in. He said he only knew Brother Tom slightly, but had heard of the great work he was doing. Obviously, Tom's reputation had spread far beyond Sarajevo and soon I was to learn that everybody irrespective of class, creed or ethnic origin held Tom in the highest regard.

I was now so tired that I would have gladly slept on the roof and made no objection. So when I thanked him profusely for the accommodation, I think he looked almost embarrassed. He then led me to the kitchen where the ginger-haired woman had a place set on the table with a loaf of coarse brown bread and some tomatoes, all ready to be eaten. I thanked her and sat down to eat. She fussed about, obviously intrigued by this foreign guest. It was probably her first time to see an Irishman. She kept busy at the sink while I ate and helped myself to coffee from the pot she had set brought me. When I was finished, she insisted on carrying my suitcase back to my sleeping quarters.

My priest friend was waiting there and said he knew I was going to Sarajevo but that it would take a few days to arrange the journey. Meantime I could go out, but not go far. 'These are dangerous times for all of us especially for strangers…and more so if they are Christians … the great majority of people who live in Zenica now are Muslim and they are suspicious of all non-Muslims especially since the attacks by the Croats.' I was learning fast. I said I needed a rest anyway and that I would be no trouble. I would attend Mass and perhaps take a short walk outside in the early morning or late afternoon until he could get rid of me.

'You are welcome to attend Mass of course' he said ' but it is better to do so from the gallery rather than arouse comment by being seen in the body of the church.' This was for real. This was no game. Informers, spies and undercover police were everywhere, even at Mass.

He then showed me another door which led via a passage way and narrow steps to the organ loft. I could attend Mass from there unobtrusively.

I thanked the quiet spoken priest once more and, after getting Mass times, retired to the office where I lay down gratefully on some sort of quilt and fell fast asleep as soon as my head hit the ground. I slept well and long and did not wake until eight o'clock next morning.

Some men called the day after I arrived and spoke earnestly with the priest, obviously about me and equally obviously about wanting to pass me on as soon as possible. I heard them mention my name a few times and, as they did, one or other would turn his head and stare at me while the others nodded gravely.

I only remained a few days in Zenica and so saw little of what seemed to me a drab place. Apart from going to Mass, my activities were few. The Bosna River was close by and I walked there on my first morning and saw the locals fishing. They seemed to catch nothing. The country 'Bosnia' gets its name from the Bosna River, so it must be good for something. Everyone who passed viewed me with curious stares. Perhaps because of my pale skin or the cut of my clothes. I do not know. But no one accosted me. I was out of place. I became paranoid and began to feel hostility everywhere.

Ethnic and religious intolerance gave the people good grounds for viewing strangers with suspicion. During the days I was there, the story went about that 35 Croats had been hanged in the square, in front of the church, because they refused to become Muslims. Although this was a fabrication, a propaganda ploy to stir up inter-faith hatred, many believed it and I was among that number. It tallied with the prevailing atmosphere of the day and with Zenica's long history of inter-necine violence.

So I think I was lucky to have escaped the consequences of a foolish ramble on my second day there. It was about 3 p.m. in the afternoon. It was hot in my 'room' and I was restless, perhaps beginning to get cabin fever already. So when things were quiet outside, body functions at their lowest, and most sensible people were having a siesta, I cautiously left the compound and walked the short distance to a small shop, close to the church, to buy biscuits and bread. It was indeed a small shop; just one man stood behind a little counter with his back to a limited stock of tinned beans, matches, cigarettes, alcohol, cheap packets of biscuits, a few old-fashioned 'rounds' of bread and general *bric-a-brac*. He glared at me and only reluctantly gave me a round of bread and two packets of plain biscuits when he saw my deutschmarks. He offered no wrapping and no paper bag, so I stuck the biscuits in my pockets and kept the bread in my hands.

There were no other customers in the shop at the time, but as I was about to leave, two tough looking Bosniaks blocked my way and asked me something in their language. I said 'Ireland ... IRA ... Bobby Sandys..., Roy Keane ... de Valera' – anything I could think of that might soften their attitude. For they were very close, in my body space, and one was fingering something in his pocket, perhaps a knife ? I could see they were hesitant, not knowing what to make of me. This gave me a chance to go. The church was barely two minutes walk away and I headed there, heart pounding and palms sweating. They stood arguing with each other and then started to follow me. I quickened my pace half-glancing over my shoulders but they were now coming closer. Thank God, I was so near the church gates.

I hurried now, almost in panic, and was expecting to be caught by the collar of my coat when the unmistakable sound of approaching trucks broke the stillness of the afternoon. This distracted my pursuers and gave me time to get indoors. I decided there and then to stay off the streets for the rest of my time in Zenica. I might have become one more statistic in the litany of the missing, and my journey would have been in vain.

It seems all the plotting with the English-speaking priest had come to a successful conclusion for, on the morning of my third day in Zenica, I was told everything was ready for my trip to Sarajevo and that I would be leaving at dawn the next day.

The Catholic Church should not be underestimated. It had been arranged that once I landed in Split (in Croatian hands)

I could make my way to Zenica (in Bosnian hands) where I would stay with an English-speaking priest who would use his contacts to get me escorted secretly, via a network of back roads, through Serbian held territory and be deposited on the top of Mount Igman (technically in UN hands).

Mount Igman overlooks Sarajevo and is known to many as the location of the 1984 Winter Olympics. It was then the site of a multimillion-dollar investment in hotels and ski-sports facilities, all of which were destroyed during the siege of Sarajevo. And this was the place where it was proposed to drop me, with the dubious expectation that I would make my own way down the mountain and into the city.

I thank them all, and Tom in particular, for not telling me in advance of the dangers that lay ahead. In the old days, we doctors never told patients of possible complications of operations or medicines. So the majority took medical care on faith and recovered or died in blissful ignorance of how lucky or unlucky they were. Nowadays, we present our patients with lists of so many possible side effects, adverse reactions and dangerous complications and make them sign so many documents waiving their rights away that they imagine disasters where none exist. So, with me, I was blissfully unaware of the dangers that lay ahead, just like the patients of old days. I never expected anything might go wrong. I just trusted everybody and paid whatever dollars I was asked. Lucky me.

A chilly mist swirled around the deserted square where the English-speaking priest said good-bye to me early next morning. We had walked briskly from St Elijahs in companionable silence, each deep in his own thoughts. My transport was waiting for me, once more an old black Mercedes. There were two men in front and so I got into the back where I was the sole occupant. I remember the seat was cold. Strange I should remember that and forget important things. But I am sure that is the way with many of us. We remember a snatch of a song, a certain smell or a word that was said by a stranger and forget the names of our classmates, the birthdays of our friends and the password to our e-mail.

So there I was, sitting unfazed on a cold seat. Facing another unknown journey. Trusting in complete strangers in a strange land. And my companions did not even speak English. However, they seemed anxious to get started and, after a brief word with the priest, we drove away using no lights. I cannot see that travelling in the dark made us safer since the engine noise was considerable and dawn was now dissolving the grey shadows of night. Perhaps it was to save the car's battery that we used no lights. Now that would make sense.

Before leaving the church, I had given money to the priest to thank him for his hospitality and to use as he saw fit among the poor of the parish. I had also given gifts to the ginger-haired woman who had met me that first evening and who fed me throughout my stay. I now handed over $100 to the driver of the Mercedes who grunted an acknowledgment but who never turned his head or indicated in any way whether he was pleased or not with the money. In fact, our trip was not long, certainly not worth $100, but the priest had suggested I give that amount.

After about 40 minutes, we entered a small village which in ordinary times would take your breath away with its cobbled streets and wooden faced houses adorned with colourful baskets of wild flowers and, finally, the *piece de resistance*, a small very old chapel topped by an ornate little dome rather like a mushroom. This village, straight out of Grimm's fairy tales, had somehow been bypassed by the war and nestled safe and secure in its own oasis of comfort, forgotten and untouched. It was to the church we went and pulled up at the back where there was a tidy-looking wooden house almost an extension of the church itself.

A dark robed Curé opened the door before we came to a halt, and bade us to come inside. My driver and his friend declined the offer and drove off as soon as I had got out with my bags in tow.

The Curé gave me a warm welcome and in addition spoke reasonable English. He was a thin cadaverous man with the ascetic face of someone who prays much and denies himself a lot. 'Please make yourself comfortable' he said as he ushered me inside. 'I have been told about you wanting to go to Sarajevo and a taxi will take you to the top of Mount Igman. He will be here about 2 o'clock so you have plenty of time to eat and rest till then.'

His little house was sparsely but comfortably furnished and I welcomed a very nice salad plus a glass of local red wine which he had set out on a table in the centre of the room. He did not join me but left to 'do his rounds' of the sick in the parish. Before leaving, he explained that I would have to pay the taxi man $100 'for it is a dangerous business' and 'very few take the risk nowadays.' So far, the day would cost me $200. Why am I so miserly?. Anyway by now I did not care how much it cost.

So once again I was alone. However, this time I must confess that time dragged after he left. I really had nothing to do but wait, and, as I was anxious to be on my way, every minute seemed like an hour. Yet when 2 o'clock came, I was taken unawares. I suppose I was in a half reverie, just sitting there looking out the window and watching birds as they landed, perched and flew off the roof of the church. I was aroused by a sharp knock on the door, which opened at the same time. A head appeared crowned with a mop of black curly hair. 'Doctor?'

I knew now I was being summoned for the most danger-ous taxi ride of my life. 'OK' I answered in the international language of assent. 'I'm ready… just a moment.' I gathered up my things, used the bathroom (when would I see one again?) and joined my black-haired taxi man without further ado. This time he was on his own so I sat in front. This time too, he was different in that he was a non-stop talker. Whether he was always so or whether it was nerves or whether he just wanted to practise his English I do not know, but in any case, he made a happy change from my last taxi men who uttered not a word.

I learned all about his family, lots about the war and lots about the dangers of the road he would take. He told me it was pretty safe to climb the mountain on this side but once on top, Serb artillery could pick anyone off should they feel in the mood. Generally, the UN sortied out from Sarajevo at the same time each afternoon so the Serbs usually stopped shell-ing then. Oh yes, I was pretty sure to get a lift from the UN if they were patrolling today, if I was in the right place, if I was there at the right time and if they decided to stop for me. 'They drive in a kind of circle' he explained 'and I will leave you where they usually start on the return leg back to the city.' This was followed by short silence. Would they patrol today I wondered. Why did he say 'usually' and not 'always'? Time would tell.

I left the taxi on what I can only describe as a mountain track just short of the summit. The trees closed in on the track from either side making me feel very safe and hidden – which of course was a myth as anyone could jump out and ambush me at any time. Indeed, it was an ideal spot to hide and pounce on an easy prey like me. Furthermore, no one would be the wiser and it is doubtful if there would be anything left of me to identify should the worst come to the worst. It was only afterwards that these thoughts entered my head. At the time, I was excited about the prospect of getting into the besieged city and, if I was anxious, it was merely because I wondered how long I would have to wait before someone came along and gave me a ride.

Also, it was lovely there. The air was soft and the insects buzzed happily in the undergrowth. Shafts of sunlight came through the overhanging foliage and lit up the dark pathway in a dappled tapestry of light and shade. There were bunches of blue flowers scattered here and there which were similar to the bluebells that grow wild at home. It was altogether a beautiful place.

I moved along until I found a nice spot under a giant tree about twenty metres from a corner. Here I sat on a convenient rock and had a clear view of the track both right and left for I was not sure from which direction my rescuers would come. I could not see Sarajevo, because trees blocked my view, but I knew it was down the other side of the mountain and probably only a few miles distant. So I waited.

My luck was in. Incredibly, within 30 minutes of seeing my taxi move back towards safety, I heard the rumble of approaching engines. Within minutes, an armed personnel carrier (APC) rounded the bend. I moved quickly to the centre of the track waving my hands rather like the fellows in airports who guide in planes as they approach the terminal building. I am not sure how they feel – will the airplane stop or will it run them down? – but I felt nervous. Would the lead vehicle stop or would I have to jump clear? Was it a Serb or a UN convoy? Perhaps it was a Bosnian one bringing guns to the city? I did not know or care very much at that point. I just wanted to hitch a ride with anyone. I would be on 'their side' whoever might come to my rescue. I just wanted to get away from this lovely place which would become anything but lovely after dark, when patrolling Serbs and patrolling Bosniaks would surely kill anything that moved.

My rescuers were French, real French, who looked like French and spoke French to the exclusion of all other languages. Their lead vehicle stopped and guns pointed directly at me. I had my hands up and was clearly unarmed but who knows whether or not I had grenades strapped to my back or in my suitcase. I think it was my greying hair that reassured them. An officer popped his head out and demanded who I was and what was I doing there.

'Je suis irlandais..Je suis médecin. Pouvez-vous me porter à Sarajevo ?'

He laughed. Perhaps at my *naiveté*, perhaps at my awful accent.

He said something like 'venez entrer en' which I took to mean get in, and so I did with alacrity.

The officer turned out to be a charming, polite and kind person. He was especially charming and polite when he heard my name was Colbert. 'Monsieur Colbért...' (he pronounced it Colbáre) and then exclaimed 'Vous avez un nom français, un nom français célèbre!' I tried to explain that it certainly was possible but unlikely that I was descended from the renowned 'Ministre des Finances de Louis quatorze'.

'Ah, Jean-Baptiste Colbert' he intoned reverently.

Unfortunately, the monetary expertise of Louis's finance minister did not apply to me nor was it relevant at that moment. The noise in the APC – it is like shaking small tin cans inside a big tin can – precluded all but shouting at each other, and anyway my French was failing fast, so I kept quiet as we gathered speed. We were leading a convoy of four and as such my vehicle was either the most or the least vulnerable to attack. The Serbs would probably take aim on the appearance of the first APC and take out the second one. I hoped.

My baggage and I were squashed into what seemed like the boot of the vehicle. It had a sloping metal roof so that I had to keep my head down all the time. Any bump and I would bang my head against the roof and this happened on several occasions. I thought of how Fr Robbie McCabe cut his head when I drove him to Turkana a few years earlier and wondered if this was fate paying me back for bumping him that day.

Meantime the officer or *capitaine* continued to shout back to me. He spoke so rapidly that I did not understand anything he said, except that I gathered I had been rescued by the *légion étrangère français*, the French Foreign Legion, and that UN vehicles had been shelled on the mountain the previous week.. I supposed that was why we were going so fast. He also indicated that it was *bonne chance* that he had stopped for me.

I could see the back of his head, which was moving from side to side all the time, I suppose watching for signs of an ambush. When he noticed that I was not responding to his conversation he stopped talking but would look back at me occasionally and grin, as if checking to see if I was still there. I am sure he wondered whether he had picked up a fool, a brave man or perhaps a deaf dumbhead. All I could hear was the clatter of our engine. I was not aware of the offensive being lodged against the UN on Mt Igman at the time. Otherwise, I am sure I would have imagined we were being shot at. Blissfully I could see nothing, but I knew we were descending fast and that we were zig zagging – I hoped this was to avoid potholes. Not bullets.

I learned later that I was crouched in the back of a Renault VAB (*véhicule de l'avant blindé*), perhaps the same one that was to plunge over the side of the track a few days later killing three US diplomats and the French driver.

Happily our trip was short and uneventful. But I was glad when we finally stopped. I got out gingerly and found I was standing on tarmac, on the runway in Sarajevo airport. We had pulled up in front of the terminal building. It reminded me a bit of Kigali. There were gaping holes in the roof and the bent steel framework was exposed in many places. The walls were scarred, puckered and singed from mortar fire and yet there remained unmistakable signs of better times such as an almost intact ad for Marlborough cigarettes and a sign pointing to the VIP lounge.

My rescuers led me to a building beside the terminal, which looked hard worn but intact. I was asked to show my ID and was able to produce the UN card that I had managed to scrounge – under false pretences – from a dyslexic guy in Caritas who printed my name as Colbret instead of Colbert. However, the truth is that people do not really examine IDs all that closely, and anyway, who but a madman – apart from cossetted politicians and diplomats – would want to go into Sarajevo at a time when everyone else was trying to escape from that hell hole.

So there I was, probably in the most dangerous place in the world, knowing nobody and carrying an identity card in someone else's name. Yet I felt secure. The good *capitaine* was still beside me, and I knew my contact, Brother Tom O'Grady, was in Sarajevo and expecting me.

Brother Tom had established himself as a sort of folk hero with the locals and seemed to be known by anyone who was important. He was a larger than life character who had been asked by Refugee Trust to establish a base in Sarajevo long before I came. Tom O'Grady was certainly an unusual person with unusual talents and unusual abilities. Everyone said so and I was to see him in action before long.

The duty officer had heard of him too and one short phone call was all he needed to confirm my authenticity. Tom would send a car for me and 'would I mind waiting at the airport an hour or so.' I expressed my thanks and sank back in the only decent chair I could find.

Tom's name had worked wonders. I was offered coffee and biscuits, which I duly enjoyed. They were not your ordinary digestive biscuits but rich chocolate-coated Belgian ones. And the coffee was strong, aromatic and satisfying. I was beginning to like Sarajevo already.

In less than two hours, a car arrived for me and I was whisked off to Tom's apartment. I saw little on the way for it was getting dark and there was no street lighting and no traffic. But I was very glad to be coming to the end of a day that I will never forget.

Tom lived and worked in an upstairs apartment in Ferhadija St which runs west-east ending at the famous Ferhadija mosque that marks the entrance to the old city. His office was small and cramped and anything but comfortable. However, its location was perfect and the rent reasonable.

A lot of people were coming and going and I was never sure of what they were doing except that many of them were looking for help for themselves or for their families. He had a local lady, Elma Bezdrob, to mind the books and both greeted me warmly. In honour of the occasion, Tom brought me out to eat. We went to a small basement restaurant with blackened out windows where the staff knew him well. Here we had fried eggs and French fries and coffee. We lingered over two beers at the end while he explained something about his work in Sarajevo.

He told me that funding from Ireland and other sources was just about enough for his basic needs and for a few small projects that he wanted to support. Central among them was the care of the blind in a building that had been destroyed by the bombing. In this work, he was aided by Dr Bassim, a local doctor whom he greatly admired. But it was Tom who got things going again and who paid for the labour and material needed to make the place habitable. He extended his aim of caring for those least able to care for themselves by setting up support groups in locations where the elderly, sick and disabled met daily. Here, in what Tom called 'Living Centres', they could exchange news (generally bad news), meet old friends, make new ones, play chess and drink endless cups of coffee in warm surroundings. Otherwise, they were condemned to lead neglected, isolated and fearful lives.

He also set up a system whereby local teenagers would bring food, water and medicine to the elderly and sick living in high-rise apartments. These apartment blocks were without water, electricity or any other basic amenity and were often up to 30 stories high. So Tom's 'runners' were a godsend to those stranded in apartments that could only be reached by laboriously climbing up interminable concrete stairways. I visited some of these during my time and more often than not had painful calves at the end of the day. I brought my medicine bag and dispensed what I could, but it was from distributing dollars and deutschmarks that had been given to me in Ireland that I got the most pleasure.

However, while both medicine and money were received gratefully, I think – I know – it was my climbing up the stairs in person and coming into their apartments to see and talk and 'be there' that was most appreciated by those I visited.

Shelling had damaged many of the apartments so that holes in the walls, blown out windows and leaky ceilings were the rule. A shelter of sorts from rain and wind was provided by packing cracks and gaps with cardboard boxes and old mattresses. One old lady pointed out specific windows in adjacent blocks where snipers regularly fired on her apartment block and on the road below. These were Serb snipers. Bosniak snipers would return fire from her block. This seems extraordinary, but it is true.

The reality of what that old lady told me was made clear to me on a later occasion. I was high up in an apartment visiting an elderly diabetic man one afternoon when bullets screamed in through the window embedding themselves in the opposite wall. I had been sceptical when he had told me that Serb snipers were operating in the next building and that was the reason that he had almost completely blocked the window with wooden planks. His bed was pushed into an alcove well out of the firing line and now I realised with horror that everything he had told me was true. I am sure they were not aiming at that old man specifically, and for sure, they were not firing at me? It is more likely that a Bosnian sniper was operating from another apartment in his block and that the gunfire was in the nature of a tit-for-tat exercise.

For the residents of those apartment blocks, on both sides of the 'divide', these shootings were a nightmare and, apart from injuring and killing people, they created a constant atmosphere of fear.

This fear was more than justified if you took a trip down 'Sniper Alley'. 'Sniper Alley' was one of the most notorious roads in the world at the time. It ran parallel to the river and led from the old town in the direction of the airport and was the main artery of the city. Snipers infested its many high-rise apartments and seemed to ply their disgusting trade with impunity. It was definitely the most dangerous road in Sarajevo during the siege. No one knows for sure how many died or were injured on this road during the siege. Some guess 600 lost their lives, others guess up to 1,000.

The city itself was eerie. There were no buses, no cars, no lights and no crowds of people hurrying home after work or going to nightclubs or movie houses or cafes. Yet there was a hum of underground life most easily heard after nightfall. A buzz of conversation and a haze of smoke could be found behind every door and behind every shuttered window in the numerous cafés and coffee shops of the old town and, it was to one of them, that Tom and I repaired each evening for the usual – a plate of (greasy) French fries and a fried egg washed down with a draft of beer or a mug of black coffee.

One of Tom's greatest achievements was to bring together people of diametrically opposite views and background. Thus, he hired Serbs and Bosniaks and non-believers without any religious preference and amazingly found that his mixed teams worked in complete harmony. Tom recognised that ordinary people, whatever their views, had one overwhelming desire which bound them together: the need for peace, harmony and forgiveness.

Tom had a retinue of locals working for him. He needed locals not only to oversee his work but also to liaise with the civil authorities and with other NGOs. Many groups gave him money or donated goods and it was Tom's genius for eloquently and persuasively presenting the needs of the ordinary people to such groups that allowed him carry out his mission. This he did in a manner that far exceeded anything one might reasonably expect or hope for. In pursuit of his aims, he attended numerous diplomatic parties and was on first name acquaintance with the Mayor as well as the Heads of most humanitarian missions in the city including the UN chiefs.

He brought me twice to visit Cardinal Vinko Puljić who persuaded me to raise funds for the roof of the Catholic Cathedral, which had been badly damaged by shelling. 'I know this is not a priority' he explained 'but when you return to Ireland perhaps you can do something about it among the Catholics there.' When I returned to Ireland, I put ads in the Catholic papers and took in a decent amount of money, which

I forwarded to the Cardinal. I was happy to see a fully repaired roof a few years later when I revisited the city in peacetime.

Life in Sarajevo

Unfortunately, my accommodation was not exactly what I would have wanted. For starters, it was across the river from the old town and so was quite close to the encircling hills where the Serbs had their gun emplacements. It also meant that at least twice a day I had to cross a bridge, which was a favourite target for snipers. There were warning signs *Pazi-Snajper* and *Beware Sniper* at both ends of the bridge – and in both languages.

These only heightened my fear when crossing it. Most times, I ran across in a half-crouching position, but I am not sure that this was actually of any benefit. Perhaps I gave the snipers a laugh. Once or twice, I thought I heard a bullet smacking into the parapet on my right or left but this was probably my overactive imagination. On no occasion was I hit. This was just as well because the Polyclinic – where the sick and injured were treated – was on the foothills on Tom's side of the river, and there was no way I could reach it in an emergency. Indeed the Polyclinic was itself a target for shelling. I spent a few mornings there and saw this for myself. Operating theatres were going day and night and the staff was tired and dispirited. There was no pay of course but government chits – IOUs – were handed out in the expectation that they would be honoured when the world came back to normal.

Everything was in short supply, particularly anaesthetics, analgesics and antibiotics. In a makeshift way – at which man is so inventive – metal coat hangers were sterilised and used as internal fixation devices for fractured limbs. That seemed to me as smart as our use of pieces of mosquito nets to substitute for expensive commercial mesh grafts in hernia repair in Africa. At the time, I wrote the following for the Refugee Trust Newsletter: 'Its World War One stuff here…the conditions in the hospital are bloody awful…They're using pieces of bayonets and copper piping as orthopaedic screws.'

A second drawback with my accommodation was that it was a one-bed apartment close to the roof of a high rise 'communist-style' apartment block. This entailed a long climb every evening, with limbs already worn out after a day of trudging around the city.

But the greatest drawback was the lack of water. I used to queue up at a communal water pump most mornings and fill a small bucket, which I carried back to my room. There were several ashtrays in my room and I would use the largest of these to wash my face and use a smaller one to wash my teeth. Thus cleansed, I would make my way down, deposit my empty bucket on the ground floor under the concrete stairs and make the journey across the river having to run the gauntlet one more time.

I understood from those who stood in line with me that the Serbs used the water queue for firing practise, almost as a sport. Civilians had been shot and killed while queuing for water and on one occasion eight people lost their lives while standing in line. As a result, we were all as quick as possible in filling our buckets and we used small containers in case we would provide too easy a target for snipers while filling large ones. Besides, water was scarce and only available at certain hours, and I do not think one would be popular with the rest of the queue if one stood there with several large buckets to fill.

There were parts of the city where water pumps were safer and this included the area near the two principal Christian churches, the Roman Catholic Cathedral of the Sacred

Heart and the Serbian Orthodox Cathedral of the Nativity of the Theotokos (Mother of God). Tom's house was fairly well shielded from shelling by these and adjoining buildings although the Roman church was definitely a target for the Serb gunners.

On one occasion, I saw two young men filling large buckets with water from one of these safer water pumps. Once full, they carried them the short distance to Tom's apartment block. I stood watching as they ascended the narrow stairway, splashing liberally as they climbed higher and higher. A few minutes later, they returned with empty buckets only to refill them and disappear inside the building once more. On enquiry, I learned that they were filling Tom's bath so that he could have a decent wash once a week! It is again strange that I should remember such a trivial thing in the midst of the grief, carnage and devastation that surrounded us on every side.

Without a doubt those young men almost idolised Tom. He had secured safe passage for whole families out of Sarajevo through his contacts. He had provided employment at a time when there was no paid work to be had. And he was generous to all. For money was not just scarce, it was gone for the vast majority who took and gave out doubtful IOUs or bartered things – often precious things – for food and fuel.

Even the army went unpaid for long periods only being provided with basic food rations, cigarettes and the uniforms they wore. Each night, groups of soldiers would leave a barracks, which was close to my apartment, and wait in dug outs and redoubts watching for enemy incursions until they were relieved at dawn. I spent a few hours one night with a group of them but apart from one false alarm all was quiet.

Nor do I think my presence was very welcome. No one spoke to me except the officer who grudgingly let me come along. In retrospect, I think they were right to be suspicious of any stranger. I think they only let me come because they knew I was a doctor.

In many ways, the succeeding weeks are a blur. Yes, I remember some individual incidents with crystal clarity, yet I would find it impossible to give an accurate day-by-day account of my short time there.

I have often thought it perverse that Ireland sometimes fails to recognise the work of those like Tom O'Grady who truly deserve to be honoured while often showering accolades and giving honorary degrees to far lesser people.

Then again, worldly honours mean little to truly fine people.

The Little Mute Girl

I have said that much of my time was spent in visiting sick and poor especially those in inaccessible or in dangerous frontline places. One such visit is etched into my mind, not because I did anything special during it, not because the person I visited was 'famous', not because I ran any special danger in the visit but simply because it touched me so deeply.

There was a small house on my side of the river across from the great library of Sarajevo which now lay in ruins. Four people lived there. A father, a mother, the mother's sister and a little five-year-old girl. They had no money and no means of support except the little we gave them on occasional visits. Tom had organised that some of his team would supply several families, including this one, with a few loaves of bread, some rice, tinned milk and a few other items every few weeks. People waited for these visits eagerly and managed to survive on what we brought them until the next visit. The team leader explained to me that the house we were going to visit had been hit by a shell the previous year but was now quite habitable. Then she went on to explain that early in the siege, when the Serbs actually made incursions into the city, some militia men had pushed down the door, knocked the father out of the way and raped his wife and sister-in-law before his eyes and before the eyes of the little girl. The father had tried to stop them but they felled him with rifle butts, kicked his prone body and shot him in the groin, mocking that he would not need his balls again. Unfortunately, some of the bullets had also severed his spine so that he could no longer walk. He had been a private in the Bosnian army. Now he was of no use to anyone.

Friends helped out, but friends too had their own worries and their own lives to consider, and so, as time went on, things got worse and worse for this little family. The first time I saw them, they were all sitting together in their semi-repaired kitchen-cum-living room. The little girl was on her mother's lap and looked at me with great suspicion. She had big black eyes that seemed to look right inside me and ask 'Why are you here? ... Have you come to hurt me?'

The team leader was one of several Serbs who worked for us and, although I forget her name, I remember well her distinctive Roman nose, her bright intelligent face, her ready smile and especially the kindness she showed to everyone. She was as moved by this family's story as I.

While she brought in the supplies, I sat down and offered the little girl some of the 'special' sweets that I kept for the little ones I met on my daily rounds.

She neither smiled at me nor answered my greeting nor put out her hand to take what I offered. It was obvious that she was afraid of this strange man. Who could blame her? All I could do was leave the sweets beside her and gently rub the little arm that clung so fiercely around her mother's neck.

We took our leave promising to be back in two weeks with more food. Once outside, the Serb lady told me that the little girl had not spoken since that dreadful day when her mother was assaulted and her father shot. She told me other stories of live babies being thrown into the river in front of their parents and of fearful reprisals, lootings, burnings and shootings being perpetrated by all sides. I had no reason to disbelieve her although I suspect many stories are exaggerated and sometimes complete fabrications..

For, like doubting Thomas, it was only what I saw with my own eyes that stuck in my brain. The image of the little girl and that sad family was to haunt me for a long time afterwards.

I made one more visit to that house before I left. It was probably a month or three weeks later and I made sure I would be with the team that afternoon. I specifically brought a black-haired doll as a gift for the little girl (I never learned her name).

This time the reception was very different. The mother was smiling, the aunt was busy cooking something over the stove and the father was doing some work with a knife, carefully paring away at a piece of wood. The little girl was playing on the floor and smiled at us as we entered. The same Serbian lady as before was with me and, after talking for a few moments to the mother, she told me that the little girl had started to speak again after our last visit.

This was a bright, lovely, precious moment for me. It was like a lighted candle in the middle of a black night. I went back to that same place a year after the siege had been lifted and met them all again. There are no words that can express the happiness of that visit nor can I begin to describe my delight at seeing the little girl chattering away and skipping with a piece of rope, just like any normal kid. I still do not remember her name. The family have moved elsewhere in Bosnia but I could find the house if I went to Sarajevo again.

Irreplaceable Buildings

As far as I could see there was not a single building in Sarajevo that escaped the shelling unscathed. Certainly, this was true of central Sarajevo and it was most marked on those lovely buildings that lined both sides of the Miljacka River.

The world-renowned Library was one of the first to be destroyed. I recall with sadness making my way through the rubble one Sunday morning and picking a path among burned books and charred tables and chairs. They say that up to three million books were lost forever. I know that brave citizens risked their lives in saving some of the rarer manuscripts. It is strange to me how all through history we have done our best to destroy anything of beauty or anything of historic importance. Wikipedia shows a picture of the 'Cellist of Sarajevo', Vedran Smailović, playing his cello in the rubble of the library in 1992. I never met him, but I am sure he anguished with the people of Sarajevo more than most, and I am also sure that he kept their spirits up during those dark days more than most.

A couple of hundred metres down the river, on the same side as the Library, stands the beautiful General Post Office, a jewel in the architectural crown of Sarajevo. It still stood defiantly upright towards the end of the siege and its empty windows stared out at the world like so many accusing eyes. It reminded me of how the Reichstag must have looked in May 1945; a gaunt empty shell, a gruesome reminder of the folly of humankind.

The third riverside building I recall is the Jewish Museum. This was pillaged by the Nazis in 1941 and was the place where Sarajevo's Jews were rounded up before deportation to concentration camps. The reconstructed museum is now located in Baščaršija (old market), on the other side of the Miljacka River, and is a major tourist attraction. The Synagogue is the oldest in the Balkans, dating from 1581. Although a target for Serbian gunners, it is surrounded by mosques and difficult to pinpoint. It suffered nothing like the damage inflicted on the Ashkenazi Synagogue situated further down on the left bank of the river.

Lastly, I must mention two bridges. The first is the Latin Bridge. This is an old Ottoman stone arch bridge that spans the Miljaka west of the General Post Office and is reputedly the oldest bridge in Sarajevo. The corner on the northern end of the bridge is the site of the assassination of Archduke Franz Ferdinand of Austria and his pregnant wife on Sunday 28 June 1914.

The whole story makes poignant reading. Only a small insignificant plaque on the corner house facing the river commemorates that fateful day.

When I stood at the spot in 1995, I felt a strange sense of futility, not just about the work I was doing but also about the future of Sarajevo itself.

The second is the Peace Bridge, known by its old name the Vrbanja bridge. It lies further out from the city centre than the Latin Bridge and was the site of the abduction of French UN soldiers by Serbian forces who fooled them by dressing in French uniforms in May 1995 just before my visit. The French reaction was swift and fearful and included air strikes on Palé a major stronghold of the attackers.

Markale Market: The Second Massacre

At approximately 11 a.m. on the 11 August 1995, I approached the Markale market. The market is situated in the old town, behind the RC Cathedral, and I was heading there to pick up supplies from brother Tom's place. I was almost there when I heard a short series of thumps that sounded like corks being popped off bottles. This was followed by the sound of screaming and then I saw that people were running towards my car, obviously away from something terrible.

It was broad daylight, the sun was shining, the orange trees in bloom and, up to now, the morning had been a typical summer Sarajevo morning. The only unusual feature was the lack of shelling from the Serb lines during the past 24 hours.

I decided to see what was happening as it was fairly obvious that anyone with medical skill might be of use. It took me only a few moments to reach the market and get out of my car. I literally fell over the first dead body. Looking around it seemed that hundreds were dead, as bodies were lying singly or in groups all over the place. But in fact, most of these were pretending to be dead and scared that more bombs would explode or that Serbs forces would come raging through any moment. Eventually it turned out that 43 had died and that less than 100 were wounded.

The market street is narrow and it was filled with overturned stalls, produce spilled everywhere, bodies lying at all kinds of unnatural angles, wounded men and women and children crying in pain, helpers fumbling around doing their best to calm the uncalmable and overall there was a sickly sweet smell.

I was of little use. I was just a foreigner telling people 'You'll be all right ... Help is coming ... Stay calm ... Don't move....' And of course few understood what I was saying. Yet there is some comfort in knowing that another human being is sharing your grief, however ineffectual words may be in bringing practical help. Later, when the road had been cleared, the bodies removed and the wounded brought to the Polyclinic, I watched as people came silently and laid wild flowers and lit small candles around each of the little craters caused by the mortar shells.

I understand now that only five shells were fired at the market that day. I understand too that they were fired – deliberately targeting civilians – by the Army of Republika Srpska – although at the time this was hotly denied by them – just as they had previously denied in a similar attack on the same place a year earlier when 68 civilians lost their lives.

The counter claims came fast. The Serbs stated that the Muslims, desperate to get the West to intervene militarily in the conflict, had fired the shells from another part of the city. That was enough to sew the seed of doubt in those who wanted to hear it.

The following Sunday I attended a memorial Mass for the victims in the Sacred Heart Cathedral. It was a sad occasion. The church was full and people of all races and all religions filled the seats. There was little talk, just an air of expectancy, waiting and depression.

There is a large stained glass rose window behind the main altar. It is a focal point of the church. On sunny days, it casts a warm red glow right down the central nave, which bathes the whole church in a luminous aura. The window itself depicts Christ hanging limp on the cross at Calvary. During some previous attack, a shell must have struck the window and torn through Christ's heart, for now there was nothing in the centre of his chest but a large jagged hole. It seemed to express how everyone felt that morning, so many hearts were broken and so many lives had a void that could never be filled.

The service was moving. The only discordant note was struck when a large black American soldier mounted the pulpit and started taking photos of the mourners. Doubtless he was unaware of the level of grief being suffered by the congregation. But somehow, it upset me greatly.

I am normally an inoffensive person and reluctant to confront others in public. On this occasion, I got up, mounted the steps of the pulpit and asked him to stop taking photographs. He seemed to suddenly realise how inappropriate his actions were and stopped immediately. He was a big guy and could have told me to go to Hell. I am glad he did not, as I could have done nothing to stop him. I expect he just wanted special photos to show at home.

August 1995

The beginning of the end came on the night of 30 August 1995. I remember it vividly. NATO planes came in waves overhead, bombing Serbian positions on the surrounding hills and lighting up the night sky with flashes that dazzled, terrified and yet exhilarated us as we waved sticks, hats, flags – indeed anything we could lay our hands on – in welcome to what we saw as an avenging ally, come to deliver us from our misery. Stupidly, foolhardy people – including myself – watched the spectacle from the roof of our buildings, never thinking that a bomb might go astray and send us to our doom. Adrenaline banishes not just fear but also reason.

Clearly, the bombing was in retaliation for the Srebrenica massacre but we did not know that, nor did we guess that full liberation would not come until 1996. Nonetheless, that night was the first time in four years that real hope was born for the beleaguered Sarajevians.

The United Nations Protection Force as they were called, had now a firm grip on things, due largely to the NATO airstrikes, which were prompted by the second Markale massacre.

The city was beginning to come to life again.

Officially the Bosnian War ended with the formal signing of the Dayton Peace Accords on 14 December 1995. But unofficially reprisal killings went on for at least another year. One way or another I was determined to go back because I knew full well that once Bosnia was no longer an exciting media story, then it would be forgotten. And media interest would move on to the next big story. Meanwhile the aftermath of years of war would continue to affect the ordinary people who had been displaced, bereaved and beggared.

I remember saying 'Never again ... Never again' at the time. How foolish. But who could have foreseen what was to befall Iraq, Afghanistan and Syria in the years that followed?

Palé

After a brief break at home, I returned to a liberated Sarajevo. This time I managed to get a trip out of the city to Palé (pronounced Pa–lay). Palé is a small town lying to the southeast of Sarajevo and was the administrative seat of the nascent Republic of Srpska. Many high-ranking Serbian officials and military commanders directed operations from there during the siege. But now, when we drove into the town, the streets were deserted and the whole place looked like an empty Hollywood set. Although we were technically safe, we felt ill at ease and did not get out of our vehicle but turned around and drove straight back to Sarajevo hardly exchanging a word.

Palé has a long and turbulent history of massacres, ethnic cleansing, sectarian pogroms, oppression of minorities, internecine fighting and political unrest stretching back beyond Ottoman times. Nowhere was the jackboot of the Nazis more ruthlessly stamped than in Palé when Yugoslavia was being dismembered in 1941.

In the process, Palé was incorporated into the new state of Croatia; all Serb businesses were shut down and the Orthodox

Church in Palé was destroyed. The local Ustaše – initially Nazi sympathisers – took over the Cultural Centre and any sign of Serb resistance was mercilessly crushed. The extreme depravity of the Ustaše paramilitaries even shocked the Nazis and provoked confrontation with them shortly afterwards.

Infuriated by the treatment of Serbs, the Chetniks, composed mainly of Bosnian–Serbs, arrived. They were equally depraved and among their recoded atrocities is the notorious Drina massacre of December 1941.

Drina Massacre

This massacre is just one episode in the blood stained annals of Bosnia. And although it is probably forgotten in the West, it is still spoken of with horror and shame in the Balkans.

It was 11 December 1941, when the Chetniks, mostly Serbs, having just taken Goražde, now entered Palé, intent on revenge and especially intent on exterminating Muslims and Roman Catholics. One of the first things they did was to burn down the local convent, the Marijin dom, and put the five nuns who lived there under armed arrest.

At this point, they taunted them sexually, insulted their religion, spat on them physically and humiliated them in every lewd way they could. Then they made them march in the freezing cold across the Romanija Mountains, all the time driving them on like animals.

One nun, an exhausted 76-year-old, could go no further than the village of Sjetlina, where she collapsed. She was then made stagger into the nearby woods. The locals looked on helpless.

Next day, they spotted a Chetnik with a rosary around his neck and it was obvious to all that the nun had not given it to him voluntarily. Once the last of the gunmen had moved out, the villagers went searching for the missing nun. They found her corpse hidden among the trees a few days later.

The other four nuns struggled on to the Army Barracks in Goražde where they were locked in a third floor room. Here they thought they were safe.

Far from it. Within an hour, a group of Chetniks broke in and attempted to rape them. All four nuns threw themselves out the window in order to avoid being raped and were bayonetted to death where they lay by officers below. The bodies were then thrown into the Drina River.

The real responsibility lay with Jezdimir Dangić, Commander of all Chetniks in East Bosnia. His consistent ruthlessness even shocked the Nazis who captured him a few months later and interned him in Germany. However, he escaped and in revenge took part in the Warsaw rising of 1944.

Ultimately, the Russians caught Dangić and handed him over to the authorities in Yugoslavia in 1947 where the Communists executed him in Sarajevo for war crimes. He was only aged 50.

Should such a thing be forgotten?

Of course not. Nor should the fact that in 1992 Serb police and militia hung people in the streets of the towns of eastern Bosnia and dumped the bodies of hundreds of men, women and children *everyday* into the Drina from the bridge at Višegrad.

The spirits of the murdered must surely have risen from the waters in protest at this holocaust. But the dead cannot intervene to save the living. That is in our hands.

CHAPTER 16

THE KOČOS

I regret now that I did not keep a diary while in Sarajevo. At the time I believed I would never forget names and places. But after these years, my memories have become blurred and names and faces have merged – even disappeared – from my conscious mind. I envy those who recall everyone they have met and who keep up contact with acquaintances and friends over the succeeding years. For me, there was just one family that I met in Sarajevo with which I still maintain contact.

This was a Muslim family, who had fled from their home in Doboj, a city in northern Bosnia and Herzegovina. Both Croats and Bosniaks fled from invading Serb forces in early 1992 and the Kočo-Mašnic family was among them. They planned to flee south, hoping to find safety in Sarajevo, but turned back because the road was being continually strafed. Their only hope of safety lay in seeking sanctuary in Catholic Croatia and so they tramped north to Zagreb. They had relatives in Zagreb and prayed that they would take them in.

They were lucky. They were received with open arms and, although the little apartment was already crowded, mattresses were put on the living room floor and the couch was turned into a bed. All had to sleep in one room.

By now they had walked over 350 km (220 miles) and were physically and mentally worn out. They had slept huddled together on the side of the road, ran wildly for safety when planes swooped down with machine guns blazing, got soaked

294 | NO TEARS LEFT

when caught in the pelting rain and performed private bodily functions in full view of passer-by. Their feet were blistered and faces unwashed but still they pressed on. They spoke little but their thoughts constantly revolved around home, business, car, savings – all lost.

Yet, in the midst of this calamity, they kept on going, like automatons. They watched out for each other and when one faltered, the rest rallied around until everyone was able to continue.

So, when they reached Zagreb and were welcomed by their cousins, their spirits rose and they began to live like human beings once again. They turned their hands to any kind of work they could get such as washing and mending clothes, cleaning windows and gutters and digging gardens, as long as they could earn a few Croatian kunas. When the money they brought with them was gone, they sold their jewellery and so had enough to tide them over the first year of their exile.

There were ten of them altogether. They were headed by Emina and her 74-year-old husband Kasim. Emina was a small, middle-aged woman dressed in black from top to toe. She carried authority easily and was clearly the leader of the family. Kasim was older, grey haired and dispirited. He smiled a lot, but it was a sad smile and he was a passive soul depending on Emina completely. Indeed, everyone in the family depended on Emina. She kept their spirits up when things looked hopeless. She made decisions; she organised the cooking and cleaning and guided them through 'thick and thin'. There are people like Emina, but they are rare.

Refugee Status

After much waiting and many disappointments, after filling endless forms and shuttling from one office to another, they were given temporary refugee status. This made a great difference to their lives for they were now provided with a small apartment of their own.

In addition, they became eligible for a handout of 'flour, pasta and rice once a month' (Emina's words) but no money. And they were not allowed to work. Yet it was this adversity that moulded them into 'a real family for the first time ever' (Emina's words again).

The Kočos were always grateful to Croatia for helping them in their hour of need. Croatia itself was a poor country and was trying to deal with an economic situation that was little less than disastrous, so it was remarkable that the authorities did so much for the thousands of refugees who sought sanctuary there.

However the 'Kočos' – as I called them for short – always wanted to go home. Emina could speak five languages and had been a teacher all her life. Her husband had managed a light engineering company and their daughter was only one year from graduating as a medical doctor. Their niece, who was with them, was a graduate in marketing and had excellent language skills. They had much to offer and since they could not work officially in Croatia it is quite understandable that they ardently desired to go back to Bosnia and Herzegovina (BiH).

I was never clear how they managed to leave Zagreb and travel to Sarajevo. But they did, and this time they were given a rather nice apartment in the centre of the city, near the railway terminus. The original owners of the apartment were Serbs and had fled from Sarajevo, probably in a manner similar to the way the Kočos had fled from their home in Doboj. Emina told me the Serbs had probably gone to Belgrade but she never met them nor did she know their names.

Back in Doboj, other Serbs moved into the Kočos house and are there to this day. Doboj is now part of the Republic of

Srpska. The Kočos would love to go back but dare not, even after more than twenty years.

While in their new home in Sarajevo the Kočos took in a young man called Demir. I am not sure if he was a relative but I do know he had been injured in the first Markale market massacre. Demir was alone in the world and was treated with great kindness by the Kočos. I am always amazed that those who have the least often give the most. Certainly the Kočos had little of this world's goods to share. I met Demir a few times but conversation was impossible since he knew no English and I know no Bosnian, so I never found out his story.

I suppose the Kočos were better off than most in that just six of them lived in the commandeered apartment. However, Kasim was always sick, Emina was now worn out from work and worry and only one of the young people – the niece – got paid work. She had approached the Canadian Mission in Sarajevo who hired her immediately, clearly impressed by her alert manner and fluent English. Her plan was to go to Canada and start a fresh life there. Who could blame her? Meantime, to her credit, she supported the Kočos. I inferred that her own parents had been killed in the war but Emina never spoke about them and I did not ask.

Emina spoke excellent French and that made communication between her and me easier. Indeed, she still writes to me in French and I reply in English, which she can read tolerably but cannot speak well at all.

My meeting the Kočos was fortuitous. Brother Tom had gone to see someone in the UN to get funds for one of his projects and I was left with a free afternoon. I still had some money left so I asked Drago, one of our local team, to bring me to any family that he felt really needed help. It took only a moment for him to suggest that we should visit the Kočos. It turned out to be an afternoon well spent. I knew that from the moment I met them.

Perhaps I focused too much on that one family, but I felt it was better to help someone properly than to waste whatever I had by spreading it too thinly around.

I promised them that I would bring my wife Doreen, and my sister Sibyl, to see them after the war. It was a promise I hardly believed myself at the time. In the meantime I sent them money which was more than matched by a volunteer group in UCG (University College Galway) headed by Gearoid OBroin, who is currently the Director of Financial Accounting in the College.

CHAPTER 17

POST-WAR BOSNIA

Sending Aid

My return trips to Bosnia were, in general, uneventful. At home we collected clothes and non-perishable food and helped fill a large container truck destined for Bosnia. Our garage was filled with black plastic bags full of donations of every kind, which we sorted diligently, and packed into labelled boxes as best as we could. Often we would find big plastic bags of second-hand clothes left outside our gate and sometimes it seemed that people were merely getting rid of things they did not want, for many of the clothes were torn or dirty.

Nonetheless people gave generously and – despite the work of sorting and packing and the smell of unwashed clothes – we were happy because we believed everything would go to people who had nothing. We even collected medicines and canned foodstuffs. Many doctors and pharmacists gave me unwanted medicine some of which were out of date but still useful. Others gave me surgical instruments and I got suture sets and dressings from the hospital, which otherwise would have been put in the incinerator.

I met the truck in Bosnia and encountered a mountain of red tape in getting things cleared. I foolishly expected that the authorities would be delighted with free donations. But no. I suppose I could have paid money to the various officials who kept demanding that more and more forms be filled and who found fault with everything I did, but I was determined not to do so.

One problem was the fact that there were opioid drugs on board. And although they were clearly on the manifest, the customs officer accompanied me to see they were personally delivered to the pharmacist in the local hospital. In retrospect I understand the official attitude but at the time it irked me greatly. So much so that I promised myself at the time that I would never become involved in transporting things to a disaster area again. It is not worth the hassle and certainly not worth the money that must be paid on border crossings, import duties and other nefarious taxes and levies.

Worst of all was the lack of control one has over the ultimate distribution of things. I certainly cannot vouch that only the needy received our donations. I had seen this problem many times before and I really do not have any answer to it.

Obviously, I was no use at managing to deliver aid by truck. Perhaps I would have become more efficient if I had stuck at it. Brother Tom managed to accept over 120 trucks filled with humanitarian aid after the war. And he never complained.

However, there was much fun and satisfaction in retracing my footsteps after the war. Things had got better as time passed and people re-adjusted to an uneasy peace, but peace nonetheless. One of my early visits was with Norman Fitzgerald, a Holy Ghost Father. Norman was from the west of Ireland, from a well-known family in Ballinrobe in Co Mayo. He had spent much of his life in Sierra Leone, mostly working as the link person between Catholic schools and the Department of Education. He was always an outgoing person, a fine rugby player in his time and a fine golfer too. Wherever he went he brought his own special sense of humour and his undoubted organisational ability. Both these qualities enabled him to achieve much during his life.

At the time he was the Executive Director of Refugee Trust. Norman was a tall, well-built person who always had a smile on his face and whose merry eyes seemed to make light of the most serious problems. He could hold himself in any society and was truly a delightful travelling companion. I think he won most people over because of his ability to be interested in what they were saying, whether it was trivial or important.

Our visit to Sarajevo was primarily to assess the work of Refugee Trust and to see for ourselves where the greatest needs lay. Bosnia was beginning to fade from public notice, but we both knew that the aftermath of any disaster lasts long beyond public interest.

We talked about this during our return journey from Sarajevo to Split and decided that we would continue to raise funds in Ireland and operate in the new BiH until the time comes when the locals could take over and our projects either became self-sustaining or had to be wound down.

Our visits were, for me, a unique chance to see places, meet people and re-live experiences that I had during the siege of Sarajevo and to go to places that I could not visit during the war.

Everywhere we went there was destruction and hardship. People were weary, and all that remained were the memories of better days and a vague hope that tomorrow would bring some kind of respite. Once again, the futility of war was strikingly obvious for ultimately there are no winners in war.

Our first visit was short but successful, and our representatives on the ground were very appreciative that we had listened to them and had taken their concerns seriously. We were left in good spirits and determined to continue supporting their work as best we could.

Brother Tom offered to drive us to the airport. This meant a long car journey from Sarajevo in BiH to Split in Croatia, but it suited us fine, as it gave us a chance to stop in Mostar where we had a small project which needed our attention. It also gave us an opportunity to visit Medjugorje where we might say a few prayers!

Mostar

It would be hard to leave Mostar out of my story not only because the people of Mostar had suffered so much during the past decade but also because we were curious to see what remained of its 427-year-old bridge, the *Stari Most* (old bridge). For centuries, the *Stari Most*, built by the Ottoman emperor Suleiman the Magnificent, spanned the Neretva River linking Christianity and Islam. The Christian Croats lived on the north side and the Muslim Bosniaks on the south side.

In 1993, Croat shelling destroyed the bridge thereby crystallised an artificial but real division between the two communities.

You can understand then why Mostar became a graphic symbol of the Bosnian War, in which its broken bridge represented the final breakdown of trust between peoples who had lived peacefully beside each other for so long.

When I first saw the *Stari Most* in the 1980s it was a single beautiful arch. Someone had once described it as a 'rainbow of hope'. When I saw it after the war, it had been reduced to two stone stumps, one on either side of the river, joined by an improvised platform made of wooden planks strung together with ropes. Only pedestrians could use it and, even then, there was some risk when the wind blew and the whole thing swung like a pendulum.

Standing in the centre I had a clear view of the stones from the old bridge lying in the water below. The water was crystal clear and I could see the dark shapes of fish darting in and between them. There was something pathetic in the sight and I wondered about those who had laboured to carve them out of solid rock and fit them together so many years ago.

I think those medieval stone masons would have been pleased to know that shortly after my visit each stone was retrieved, numbered and re-used in restoring the bridge to just as it was in the time of Suleiman. And so it stands today in its former glory. The completed work was officially unveiled on 23 July 2004 and you would never guess that it had been a mass of rubble a few years earlier.

Norman and I only spent two days in Mostar. On the first morning, we visited the hospital and marvelled at how doctors and nurses could do such excellent work in such terrible conditions. Supplies from overseas were now pouring in and everyone we met thanked us over and over again for the help that Ireland, the United Kingdom and the United States were giving them. We accepted the thanks, as if we were personally responsible for everything.

Next day we went to the Muslim quarter where Refugee Trust had a small office. Here we met our local employees who explained how they were spending our money on supporting bombed-out families and we left satisfied that the money was well spent.

We got the sense too that all the people now wanted was peace. Just peace.

Thank You Trees

Brother Tom drove us the following day to the airport in Split. Correction. He almost drove us to Split. Let me explain. I sat in the back, Norman sat in the front passenger seat and Tom took the wheel.

We were a happy trio when we set off. The visit had been good, Tom was completely in control of his job, which was much easier now that the war was over, and both Norman and I were very happy with the way our projects were being run.

We must have been about twenty miles from the airport, with plenty of time in hand, when we approached a bend rather too fast. It was not a sharp bend, just a gentle but definite curve rounding a hill on the left. There was a deep ravine on the right-hand side. The whole area, both right and left, was covered with tall pine trees. It was truly a Transylvanian scene where you could easily imagine Dracula and his red-eyed steeds rattling along on some evil mission.

These were my boyish daydreams as we too rattled along. And rattled at speed. Some inner voice told me to open my eyes. I instinctively knew we were approaching the corner far too fast and I knew immediately we could not make it. Tom also knew as he braked desperately causing us to skid headlong towards the ravine on our right. The laws of physics prevailed. We sailed over like an arrow and bang into the waiting outstretched arms of the nearest pines. The old Land Rover did a half somersault and we settled sideways in the fork of two adjacent trees. I am certain this saved our lives.

Everything seemed to occur in slow motion, yet everything was over in the blink of an eye. The trees were so close together and their branches so intertwined that they seemed to be waiting to catch us when we zipped over the edge of the road.

Within moments, the Land Rover was quite steady as it finally sunk into its leafy parking place.

My immediate problem was a heavy weight on my chest. Norman and Tom had both been thrown backwards so that they finished up on the back seat with Norman on top of me.

We were like two cushions one on top of the other but, extraordinarily, none of us was hurt other than being a bit dazed.

I am not clear on exactly how we got out, but one by one we clambered out the rear door and scrambled up to the safety of the road. We sat on the edge and took stock. Having confirmed that none of us had a serious complaint – apart from Norman's shoulder which was bruised – we decided to hail down the next car that passed. We would leave Tom to take care of the Land Rover while Norman and I would hitch a lift to the airport.

Luck smiles on the foolish. Within fifteen minutes, a likely looking car pulled up beside us, and the driver, a young man, rolled down the window and asked us in English if we were alright. Luck smiled on him too. He and his companion, another young man, were thrilled to get 100 deutschmarks for carrying Norman and I to the airport. They clambered down to the Land Rover and retrieved our backpacks and off we went. We even had time for a coffee in the departure lounge before boarding our plane home.

I suffered no ill effects from this incident but Norman had a pain in his back for some years afterwards. Tom got the Land Rover hauled up safely and, for all I know, it may be chugging along somewhere in the heart of the Balkans to this day.

My next visit to Sarajevo was with my wife Doreen and my sister Sibyl. This was to be a real treat for them. I was anxious to show them where I had worked and had them meet the friends I had made, in particular Emina and her family. We flew in to Zagreb since civilian flights into Sarajevo were still not possible. And while in Zagreb we visited those relatives of the Kočos, who had first sheltered them when they fled Bosnia. They put on a great spread for us but it was obvious that they were far from wealthy. Their apartment was in the upper reaches of a drab block of apartments. Luckily the lift was working, and we did not have to climb endless concrete steps to reach them.

We stayed that night in the Hotel Park, which, at the time, was a dreary place with colourless dark rooms and noisy plumbing. We were glad to leave next morning and following instructions from Emina's relatives we caught a tram, which brought us directly to the Central Bus Station.

I had tried buying bus tickets from Zagreb to Sarajevo the previous evening, but this was not possible so we arrived almost two hours before the scheduled departure time. I have been caught out too often by arriving at a bus depot close to scheduled departure time only to discover my bus had left early.

Neither Doreen nor Sibyl had ever used public transport in other than a well-developed country before. Croatia was barely out of the throes of a vicious war and public services were unreliable and expensive. However our bus was already there when we arrived and there was a queue of people waiting to get tickets. Within moments there was a rush to get seats, but I was prepared for that and unashamedly pushed my ladies ahead of me and got the best seats near the front.

It was in this atmosphere that three of us sank gratefully into threadbare seats in a rather bedraggled looking bus on a grey misty morning in Zagreb and headed south towards Bosnia. We made reasonable progress but the bus was slow, very slow, and we made several stops and took several detours so that the journey dragged on interminably. The countryside was uninteresting and no one was in a mood to talk or read. We just sat there and closed our eyes, each with his or her own thoughts.

Before we reached the border, we stopped for lunch and toilet break. At this stage, the bus was three-quarters full so there was much bustling and shuffling and pushing as people tried to get out all at once. We waited our turn patiently and were rewarded by a clear walk down the centre aisle and an easy descent to the ground where the bus driver helped the ladies alight.

The bus had stopped outside a shabby building that proudly proclaimed itself 'Hotel Bosnia'. There was no other building in sight and we wondered how the owners could make a living in such an isolated place. However, our need to use the facilities was paramount and we located the Rest Rooms by the long queue waiting outside a small wooden shack at the side. Men and women were segregated. However, most men ignored the queue and did their business in the bushes behind the hotel. It was much more difficult for the ladies.

Doreen and Sibyl told me that when it was finally their turn to enter the shed, they were assaulted by myriads of flies all either going to or returning from feasting on human excrement that had not managed to make the long drop. They were then assailed by a smell of faeces and of other decaying materials that wafted up in nauseating waves from the hole in the ground, over which all users would crouch. Finally there was no toilet paper, no soap, no towel and no water in the cracked hand basin.

For my wife and sister, this was the first encounter with a long-drop latrine, and it was something they spoke of and giggled about long afterwards.

Not many were going the whole way to Sarajevo so that by the time we reached the border, there were only five people left on the bus and, I think, all but one were foreigners like us.

Formalities were brief and the examination of our passports and luggage was perfunctory. We could have been carrying nuclear bombs in our suitcases for all the bored border guards cared.

It was dusk when we rolled into Sarajevo. Tired, thirsty and grubby. We stopped at the bus terminus beside the main railway station. This had been badly damaged during the war. Lines of railway carriages, some without roofs, most without windows, and all rusting, stood forlornly on iron tracks that were fractured and twisted. But there was plenty of life about and we had no difficulty getting a taxi.

Our lodging, a small convent in the old town, was at the top of a short but very steep hill. However, the taxi man deposited us at the foot of the hill stating reasonably that his old car could go no further. He took our deutschmarks quickly enough but declined the chance of earning more when asked to carry our cases by saying he had a bad back.

We were tired and sticky and I shall not easily forget the three of us pulling our heavy loads up that hill. We had to walk in Indian file because the street was so narrow and we were silent because we had no spare energy to talk. The convent looked like any other house, and I was afraid I would miss it. I hoped I did not transmit my apprehension to the ladies for I am sure they trusted in me completely. We were almost at the top of the hill when I recognised the polished brass doorknob on the convent door. A palpable wave of relief appeared on my companions' faces when I announced that this was the convent at last.

The convent was as I had remembered it during the war. Spotless and quiet, but this time it was filled with the scent of fresh flowers from the convent garden. A young nun answered my knocking and showed us to our rooms which were small but more than adequate.

After a short time, she returned and led us downstairs to the refectory where there was a spread of sandwiches and an electric kettle to make tea. She then bade us goodnight and told us there would be Mass in the morning in the convent church at 8 a.m., if we wished to go there. She also told me that, in our case, there was no charge for the rooms.

It is only in recent times that the stories of atrocities against catholic nuns and priests carried out by Bosnian Serbs and Bosnian Muslims have become common knowledge. Many of these accounts were so horrifying that Pope Francis, visibly moved, tore up his prepared speech when visiting Sarajevo in 2015 and spoke off the cuff of his distress and of the need for forgiveness.

It is always good to show those you love where you have worked, to let them meet people you know well, to have them soak in the atmosphere of a place that is deep in your own psyche, even if it is alien to them. So it was on our visit to Sarajevo. Foremost of such sharing was our meeting with the Kočos and the unbounded joy with which they received us. My ladies soon forgot all about Hotel Bosnia and the bus ride from Zagreb.

The Kočos were in the same apartment near the railway station, but now it was warm and tidy and more like a home. Emina cried on seeing us. I suppose she remembered the dark days of the siege when I first met her and my promise to come back one day with my wife and sister. And now it was different. There was beer, soft drinks, sandwiches and cake – all that they could give us as if to say 'Thanks for not forgetting your promise'. They spoke little of the war. Instead they spoke of 'going home some day to our own place'.

I thought it is as well to let them keep this dream.

We returned to Dublin happy in the knowledge that, despite its small size and despite its many shortcomings, Ireland had played some part in fostering reconciliation between Croatians, Bosniaks and Serbs. Let us hope this reconciliation will last and be a beacon of hope for those places where differences are only settled by violence.

CHAPTER 18

Kosovo

It was June 1999, four years after the official end of the Bosnian War. Unfortunately, fresh trouble had erupted in Kosovo and once again there were murders, revenge killings, pillage and mayhem. Overt ethnic cleansing resulted in streams of people leaving Kosovo to seek refuge in other lands. The initial trickle turned into a long procession of weary families trudging the roads in search of someplace to lay their heads and in search of someone to give them food and shelter.

It is a familiar story, repeated over and over again in the history of mankind. But no amount of repetition should harden us to the terrible suffering refugees endure. Economic arguments crumble to dust when you actually see the agony in the faces of those who stumble along, all with pathetic loads on their backs, some pushing hand carts in front of them and others carrying infants or helping old people. All they seek is a future. For their past is gone.

So once again I agreed to visit the Balkans on behalf of Refugee Trust.

This time I went to Montenegro. Access to Kosovo was difficult and dangerous, and besides, Refugee Trust was supporting refugees in a large UNHCR refugee camp near the Montenegrin city of Bar. The Camp was called Neptune, perhaps because Bar lies on the Adriatic sea.

Refugee Trust employed a small team locally to administer its funds and we wanted to be certain that the money given by the donation-weary people at home was being well spent. I also had an ulterior motive in that many people had given me money, which they wanted spent 'as I saw fit'. For me, that meant physically putting money into the hands of the most needy people. So I had to get on a plane and go there.

Our two-person team, a local woman Marica Tančič and an Italian man, Enrico Barisonzi, welcomed me. It did not take long to see they were both good people and completely committed to helping the refugees as much as they could.

Enrico was a young man who spent his time going to different families and seeing what he could do for them. He loved children and was always followed by groups of little ones with whom he sang songs and played games. He reminded me of the Pied Piper, for he often headed a procession of dancing children as he went from tent to tent.

Marica was the administrator and kept a note of every penny she received and saw it was spent wisely. She was also responsible for hiring and firing local help. It was her steady hand rather than the Italian's impetuous head that kept the show on the road.

I was delighted to see the contrast between the refugee camps in Montenegro and the ones I had seen previously in Ethiopia, Kenya and Biafra. My first impression was that the tents were spacious, neat, orderly and clean. There was sufficient space between individual tents to allow children to play and provide some sense of dignity and privacy for the inhabitants. Although cooking was communal, it seemed to me that the quality and quantity of the food distributed was excellent and I was assured that the vast majority of people believed – rightly as it turned out – that they would be re-patriated in the coming months.

A Japanese UN official took overall control of the operation and we would gather at his conference each morning to agree a plan for the coming day and the week ahead.

Discussion, agreement and action were the three elements on which we worked so that each NGO knew what exactly to do. This avoided overlap, confusion and mixed messages, and allowed the NGOs to contribute according to their individual capabilities. Refugee Trust was asked to take care of waste disposal and sanitation and, while this was not a glamorous assignment, it was a very important one.

As a freelance, so to speak, I wandered around the camp, went into tents, spoke to people and gradually gained their trust and soon began to understand their grievances, worries and frustrations. I got to know that several families very well, simply because I had the time to spend with them. All their stories were moving and all were united in their desire to return to their homes in Kosovo as soon as possible. There was a surprising lack of bitterness in their accounts of how they had been treated and this impressed me more than anything else.

But this sanguine view merely expresses how things were for some of the families I met. Things were different for others as an extract from what I wrote at the time clearly demonstrates:

'...in Camp Neptune, not too far from the port city of Bar, we have only 10 toilets for 5,000 people. Can you imagine the stench in the summer heat? The stories of individual people are sad and true. I know this because I wandered around freely and spoke to hundreds of people during my visits. Many had walked from Kosovo – 300 km – carrying their bits and pieces. Some carried deformed children. Others helped the old and infirm. The television we see is somehow sanitised and unreal. You get neither the grime, the heat, the rain nor the numb despair that is really there. Many – including men – wept openly when I gave them money. They told me they were given only 5–10 minutes to get out of their homes and during that time they grabbed whatever valuables they could and left.'

Why Me?

This is the story a 16-year-old boy told me one afternoon when I entered his tent and found him sitting with his parents.

He told me they had left their house in fear for their lives and had joined the thousands of refugees who were now slowly moving along the road out of Pristina.

After just an hour his mother felt weak and, spotting a house well in from the road, they decided to ask the people if they could rest awhile. They got no answer to their knocking and thinking that the house was empty they went around the back and surprisingly found the back door open. They went inside and found themselves in a kitchen which had been clearly ransacked, for everything was in disarray, with chairs overturned and crockery smashed on the floor. The humming of a fridge in the corner told them that there was still power, but more importantly they thought there might be some food in it, for they were hungry. The son opened the fridge and suddenly screamed with pain. It had been booby-trapped with a grenade and, before their eyes, the boy's hand was blown off.

Somehow they stopped the bleeding and continued their journey to Montenegro, begging as they went and supported by others who had brought food and money.

Helping this boy became a bit of an obsession with me. He told me several NGOs had promised him a new arm, photographed him from every angle, and then, after promising him a new arm had gone away never to be seen again.

He looked at me with eyes that said 'Why me?' and I had no answer.

It is hard to blame him for being sceptical when he met me, yet another do-gooder, taking photographs and measurements and promising him the same thing that he had ben promised so often before. I determined that I should not let him down like all the others.

Thanks to the generosity of people in Ireland and the United Kingdom we succeeded in getting him a replacement arm a few years later. I have not seen him since but have been told he is very happy with his new arm.

Collateral Damage

This is a euphemism that military people use but which is of little comfort to those affected. I did not see any myself but on observing NATO planes returning from air strikes in Kosovo, and discharging unused ordinance on the border mountain ranges, I asked locals what was happening.

They told me that the planes were not allowed to return to the aircraft carriers with unexploded bombs and had to dispose of them safely before they landed.

Then they added that mountain dwellings had sometimes been inadvertently hit in these missions and, in one case, that a mountain monastery had been hit. Collateral damage.

This angered me a lot. So much so that when I went to Sarajevo a few weeks later I stopped two uniformed US soldiers in the street and bitterly accused them of killing civilians. I told them they were hated by all of us. The soldiers, one black and one white, stood numbly in front of me and said nothing.

I had released my anger like an exploding pressure cooker and felt relieved. But now I feel ashamed. Those poor fellows were thousands of miles away from home and stuck in a place where they were liable to be spat at or even shot. And they meant to do no harm; they only meant to do good.

On my next visit – which was in winter 2000 – I went further and penetrated Kosovo itself. This time Bernadette McKenna, from Refugee Trust's Dublin office, accompanied me.

Bernadette was originally from Monaghan town, but had lived with her sister in Dublin for a long time, and spoke with a rather soft north city accent. She had worked in the Bank but had always wanted to work at something where she could help people directly. So she left the Bank and went to work with Fr Norman Fitzgerald, in Refugee Trust, at a much lower salary.

She was 30 something when I met her, single, attractive and always smiling. It is a cliché to say that everyone loved Bernadette, but a cliché is a cliché because it is true. Everyone did love Bernadette. Certainly, both Doreen and I loved her.

Yet she had never physically seen any of our projects. I felt this was a mistake. She could surely talk to people about the work of Refugee Trust with much more authority if she spoke from personal experience.

Consequently, I often said to her 'Bernadette you must come and see the actual projects for yourself – as they really are. Reports never give you the true picture.' Eventually she did come.

It was winter and Dublin was unseasonably cold. But when Bernadette and I left, we knew that Kosovo would be far colder. For that reason we both brought heavy winter coats and lots of socks and strong walking boots. We foolishly believed these would keep us warm but were soon disabused of this notion when we faced one of the worst winters recorded in Kosovo in recent times.

However ignorance is bliss and we departed Dublin in good spirits, although Bernadette was slightly uneasy as to what might lie ahead. I knew Bosnia and Sarajevo very well and had visited Montenegro that summer. Bernadette knew none of these places and neither of us had ever been to Kosovo, or Transylvania as I called it. The only image I had of the latter was of a land covered with forests and inhabited by wolves and redolent with stories of vampires.

We landed first in Sarajevo. The airport showed all the scars of the war but functioned well and was now open to limited civilian traffic.

We stayed in the same convent, at the top of the same hill, where I had stayed on my previous visit. I thought the nuns eyed me curiously since they had not seen Bernadette before. Not that I blame them should they have been suspicious. Morals were notoriously low in Sarajevo, not least because of the presence of UN soldiers who could offer money, protection and jobs – and sometimes even marriage – to desperate locals. But I think their suspicions were somewhat relieved when they saw the two of us at early Mass next morning.

After a day or two visiting projects in the city we drove southwest towards the Adriatic Sea, visiting Mostar and Medjugorje on the way. Signs of the war were everywhere. Towns and villages were in ruins, and even isolated farmhouses had been destroyed. Churches and mosques were obviously special targets and we hardly saw an intact one as we drove along the narrow icy roads.

The weather stayed bright and cold but, apart from the odd flurry of hail, there was no major snowfall. In a heated car and with lots of heavy clothes we were warm and cosy as we sped past snow-covered hills, gleaming lakes and snow-laden fir trees that sparkled like jewels in the winter sun.

After reaching the Adriatic, we turned south and crossed into Croatia arriving into Dubrovnik in the early afternoon. The road we were on runs parallel to the Adriatic and when you look down you get a spectacular view of the old walled city and the sea. You have to turn off the road and descend steeply to reach the old city, and I am sure that many a car has skidded to its doom when trying to negotiate the sharp bends – even in summertime. Mark, our driver, was fully aware of this and we descended slowly and carefully without mishap ultimately arriving at sea level.

It was early afternoon when we entered Dubrovnik and the city looked its best in the crisp winter sunshine. I insisted we take time off to visit the old city and so the three of us – Bernadette, Mark and I – got out of the car and walked towards the huge walls.

There is something magical about seeing a work of art – whether man-made or natural – for the first time, and both Bernadette and I shared a magic moment as the massed walls loomed ahead of us. I did not have to ask her. We both just knew. Although Dubrovnik was a protected site since 1970, it had come under attack in 1991 by Serb and Croatian forces and it was later bombarded heavily from the sea. Despite this, the age-old walls withstood the shells and bombs remarkably well. Any damage sustained was quickly repaired and I understand that today a visitor will see nothing of the rubble or craters or shell holes that were evident on our visit.

After an afternoon of tramping around the cobbled streets, drinking coffee in a sidewalk cafe and viewing the Adriatic from the ramparts, we continued our journey. Our car, despite having four-wheel drive, strained and spluttered as we climbed back up the hill to the main road, but once there, we sped easily south towards the border with Montenegro, all the time passing magnificent vistas of sea, cliffs and islands on our right-hand side.

Twenty kilometres from Dubrovnik we stopped at a roadside inn and booked in for the night. We all slept comfortably in well-heated rooms after enjoying a good homely dinner given by the proprietor and his wife, who were very pleased to have us – their only guests in the last two weeks.

Next day we drove to the border. The scenery was as beautiful as ever and if anything the Adriatic sparkled brighter and was a deeper blue than on the previous day. Bernadette and I were happy and talkative but our driver seemed to be getting quieter and quieter as we approached Montenegro. He kept fumbling with his mobile phone sending texts and receiving calls. When we asked him if everything was ok he barely answered.

We knew we were approaching the border when we saw a long queue of trucks, cars and buses ahead but, instead of joining them, our driver came to a stop, made a three point turn and faced the car back towards Dubrovnik.

He then explained that he could not take the car across the border because it was not registered properly. He also explained that the car would be searched and anything of value taken by the border guards on both sides. Although his English was not perfect his meaning was clear.

'It easier walk across.' Our faces fell.

'It quicker, actually.' He pointed to the long queue in front of us.

'We be here ... maybe tomorrow ... before we pass.'

I knew he was right.

'But how will we get to Bar?' I asked. The town of Bar was at least a 30-minute drive from the border. Before leaving Dublin, we had contacted our representative in Bar who had promised to get us accommodation there while she organised transport to Kosovo. It all seemed to be un-ravelling now.

'Don't worry ... I phone Yūsuf. You wait other side. He pick you. He have car.' He grinned for the first time, 'Yūsuf ... he know Refugee Trust well ... he my cousin.'

I had the urge to correct him and say 'Don't say *he my* cousin...say *he is my* cousin', but then he might think I was claiming Yūsuf as a cousin of mine and the confusion would know no end. Everyone in the Balkans seemed to have a cousin when they needed one.

I now understood why he had spent so much time on his phone in the last half an hour. He had obviously been talking to Yūsuf.

There was nothing for it but to do as he said. We both had official IDs (mine still the out-of-date UN one) and I had most of our money in a canvas money-belt around my waist. Our biggest problem was carrying the suitcases, which we changed from hand to hand when one shoulder began to ache more than the other.

It was cold and crisp but the sun was shining and we even began to sweat a little as we approached the Croatian Customs and Immigration building. But we passed through this easily and had our passports stamped by a very courteous official, who wished us a pleasant trip. In ten minutes we were outside again.

Then followed the 100-metre stretch of no-man's land between the border posts. We made a lonely pair as we trudged towards the Montenegrin Immigration huts. They looked threatening and unwelcoming even in the midday sunlight. Two sullen border guards met us with guns slung carelessly over their shoulders. They bustled us peremptorily into a sparsely furnished room where we were interrogated as to who we were and why we were going to Montenegro. We were taken separately, no doubt to ensure we spoke the truth and no doubt to trap us should our stories not completely agree.

There is a sense of isolation in these kinds of places that is hard to explain. You are conscious of everything from the buttons on the official's tunic to the spider trying to climb up a dirty window, to the clock on the wall where the hands are stuck forever at five minutes past four. And most of all, you are conscious of the guards looking at you, thumbing your passport and exchanging remarks between themselves.

But once again things were in order and we were set free in just over an hour, admittedly what seemed an interminable hour. We were very happy to pay $200 border tax – in cash – get fancy stamps on our passports and walk away with all our possessions intact except for my camera, which somehow got 'misplaced' while they rummaged through my suitcase. Although I was understandably annoyed at 'losing' my camera, I showed no emotion. It was a small price to pay for getting through so quickly.

It was now afternoon and getting chilly. A cold breeze had sprung up quite suddenly from the sea and so we zipped up our coats as far as possible to protect our faces from the chill. We walked for about five minutes from the border post and sat on our cases and waited for Yūsuf. Neither of us knew him but I had no doubt he would know us. The minutes turned into hours and the sun now started to sink slowly beneath the western Adriatic, painting the clouds with an array of colours – green, purple and orange.

We gradually became not only cold, but also hungry and thirsty. Bernadette had some mint sweets, which helped a bit, but what we really wanted was a hot drink. I think being with someone gave both of us a strength that we would not have had were either of us alone.

Now the clouds changed slowly to grey and the shadows of early evening began to lengthen and creep across the road. Our conversation was desultory and pointless but still we scanned the road to Bar for some sign of a car. Quite suddenly a car approached from the south and instinctively both of us stood up and waved it down. It pulled up in front of us. It had a taxi sign on the roof and I was ready to pay handsomely to get to Bar. For some reason I imagined the driver was Yūsuf and greeted him by that name, but he shook his head saying 'Yūsuf behind … his car … no good …. He ask me to meet you.'

At this point I did not care where Yūsuf was but opened the back door for Bernadette, piled in our suitcases and went around to the front to sit beside the driver. Before he started up I got him to give me a price for the journey to Bar. It seemed high, but I was in no mood to haggle. We were tired and hungry and would have paid twice the amount he asked. Afterwards we discovered that the price he charged us was the correct one.

We clambered in gratefully and since normal conversation was difficult we just sat in silence letting him drive us wherever he wanted. We were approaching Bar when we saw a car on the side of the road ahead. The hood was raised but we could see that someone was bent under it, tinkering with the engine.

Our driver stopped, got out and approached the man who straightened up and turned around towards him. They recognised each other immediately. The man in distress turned out to be Yūsuf. Our Yūsuf. His car had broken down on the way to meet us and the poor fellow was distraught. We all got into the taxi leaving Yūsuf's car where it stood and continued without mishap into the town of Bar.

It was dark by now and the few streetlights that worked gave us little idea of where we were going except that we were heading in the direction of the sea.

Yūsuf spoke good English and told us we were going to stay in the only decent hotel in Bar – I think it was called the Villa Jadran. He also said he would collect us next day around noon, after retrieving his car.

The back of the hotel faced the beach so that guests had their own private entrance to the Adriatic. But even in good times few tourists came to this little known part of the Dalmatian coast and this was reflected in the sparseness of the facilities compared to what you find in similar resorts in the Algarve or the Costa del Sol, such as changing rooms, sunshades, ice cream parlours and the like.

Inside was no better. Our rooms were bleak but clean and each had a small heater which gave out enough heat to let you know they were working, but not enough to heat you. Furniture and plumbing were of the cheapest mass-produced kind and the paintwork on the doors and walls was flaky and faded. You locked the bedroom door with a big old-fashioned key and there was a bolt inside, which I slid across for added protection. However, the staff were friendly and courteous and, most importantly, many spoke English. I suppose that it was easy for them to be attentive to us. We seemed to be the only guests in the hotel.

Next morning we had breakfast together and even Bernadette, the most uncomplaining of companions, found the two lumps of cheese and two slices of hard black bread difficult to eat. A little butter would have helped but there was none available. However, we did get a saucer full of hardboiled eggs and we demolished these with relish. The salt was damp and lumpy and you had to extricate it by pulling the rubber bottom out of the saltcellar.

We spent the morning looking out to sea and sitting in the dreary lounge doing nothing. The only interlude in the monotony was when a lady, Anje Kapichic, came in selling her paintings. I bought one, which I later framed and called *Kosovo Cries*. Those who see it say it reminds them of *The Scream*. I would not swop my painting for Munch's masterpiece for any money.

It was afternoon before Yūsuf returned. Yes, he had the car back but no, it would be too unsafe to drive it to Kosovo.

He would hire one and have it ready for next day. Would that suit?

Bernadette and I had no choice but to ask him to make sure the next car would be a good one 'even if we have to pay extra'. He assured us that his friend had a really good car and we left it at that. He also asked us to visit his home and have dinner there. We accepted gratefully knowing that dinner in the hotel would be pretty awful if breakfast was anything to go by.

We whiled away the day doing nothing. There was lots of coffee and dry biscuits and we both had novels to read. Yet we were both very happy when Yūsuf came to collect us around 5 p.m. in yet another car. It was but a short drive to his house but again darkness had descended and we saw nothing of Bar.

His home turned out to be a cottage, and in summer it must have looked very pretty with its shrub-bordered pathway and a profusion of roses climbing up the whitewashed walls. Now it was simply a peasant's cottage something like one might find in the Scottish highlands or in Connemara 50 years ago. A hand-painted sign nailed to the front door proclaimed it to be the office of *Refugee Trust Irelande* and I am sure this gave Yūsuf added prestige in the local community.

It suddenly dawned on me that Refugee Trust had a network of employees in the Balkans all of whom were probably related to one another. My memory clicked another notch and I recalled seeing the name Yūsuf in reports from Montenegro. I then remembered that Alicja, our representative there, had rented office space in the house of a man named Yūsuf and had assured us that Yūsuf was an honest and reliable man who would take care of us in her absence for she was away when we arrived. At least we were now putting faces on people that up to then had merely been impersonal names on paper reports.

Yūsuf's wife, a small stocky middle-aged woman with a round face and a sometime attractive turned-up nose, greeted us with a broad smile and several kisses on the cheek. I could smell cooking in the background and doubtlessly she was preparing a special meal for her guests. I hoped it might be fish as there should be no shortage of fresh fish when living on the coast of the Adriatic. But we would have to wait several hours before we ate. First Yūsuf offered us vodka – which we politely refused – and then he showed us into a side room, the office of Refugee Trust.

The office consisted of a small table on which there was a sheaf of papers and a few ballpoint pens. There was a locked cabinet in the corner in which Alicja kept her accounts, receipts, chequebook and notepaper. I wondered what rent Yūsuf was charging Refugee Trust but somehow he adroitly avoided giving us a straight answer. It seems it was all lumped together with heating, light and local taxes. In the end we dropped the subject in case he would demand more.

Bernadette spent the next two hours going through the accounts and told me afterwards that they were all in order. I went for a walk to pass the time but it was cold and dark outside and I returned quickly. I was also afraid I would lose my way. When I came back, the two of them were still poring over papers covered with figures that were incomprehensible to me. I was therefore glad when Mrs Yūsuf announced that dinner was ready at last.

We were given the best places at the table. Yūsuf quickly filled my glass with home-made red wine but Bernadette refused and opted for orange juice instead. I would have insulted my hosts had I not taken their wine. Then came the main meal. Yes, it was fish, but not as I expected it. Instead we were each given a large tureen of fish stew. It was very oily and you could see onions floating about, in between the chunks of fish.

You ate the stew using a spoon but we were given a plate laden with large slices of bread, which we could dip into the stew or use as scoops to pick up the more solid bits. Yūsuf kept refilling my glass with wine. I had made the mistake of saying it was very good initially and obviously he was so pleased with my praise that he wanted me to finish the carafe.

Over dinner, Yūsuf explained that in addition to working in the office, his main job was to see that refugees from Kosovo got safely on the ferry which sailed daily to Bari in Italy. To do this, he and Alicja had to document each group, make sure their papers were in order, give them enough money to cross to Italy and distribute food and clothes parcels, as they felt fit. There were reception camps in Bari to register everyone, most of whom had been stripped of passports and money by the Serbian authorities before they fled. If all this sounds familiar, I am not surprised.

Alicja and Yusuf's jobs were difficult but satisfying. It would have been easy for them to abuse their positions. However, their records were meticulous and we never had any cause to doubt their integrity. They both knew that we would have no hesitation in replacing them if we were not satisfied.

We ended dinner with brittle sugary biscuits and thick black sweet coffee. This was served in small cups with no handles and is a favourite in the East. But I do not relish or appreciate it, so I made do with hot black tea instead.

Yūsuf brought us back to our hotel immediately afterwards, advising us to go to bed as soon as possible so that we could face the rigors of the next day's journey fully refreshed. He promised to collect us at 8 a.m. sharp.

My stomach and I slept separately that night.

Yūsuf was true to his word. There he was, at five minutes to eight, as large as life, sitting grinning in a familiar looking vehicle. The vehicle was packed with supplies leaving just enough room for the three of us. It looked like his friend's taxi.

It suddenly dawned on me. It was his friend's taxi.

'Hey Yūsuf … that is the car your friend picked us up in the other night?' I knew the answer before he answered.

'This is a good car … I promise you … See for yourself.' He got out and stood there looking admiringly at the vehicle as if that would convince us. I knew there was little I could do but accept his word. Bernadette did not seem to mind. She merely opened the back door and got in while Yūsuf and I put our cases on the front passenger seat. There was no room in the boot. At least Bernadette and I would have the whole back seat together and not have to sit on our luggage.

And so we settled down as comfortably as we could, happy that we were now embarking on the real purpose of our mission. We were now on the road to Kosovo.

Our destination there was the city of Peć (pronounced Pech), where Alicja had rented a house in which she planned to open a food and clothes distribution centre. But to get to Peć from Bar in winter posed a problem. Yūsuf informed us that many of the roads to Kosovo were impassable because of ice and snow and that some were closed by the military. However, he was going to bring us by the Čakor Pass, a mountain route, which he was reliably informed was still open. He added that it was almost certainly free of road blocks and that few travelled that way in winter apart from locals who used packhorses.

He seemed unconcerned and since we had no choice in that matter, we made no objection to his plan. I had never heard of this Pass but now I will never forget it.

The usual and best-known route to Peć (Serbian) or Peja (Albanian) is via a fairly decent road that leaves Montenegro at the border town of Rožaje. Unfortunately this road was unsafe with almost daily reports of bands of brigands hijacking vehicles and murdering their occupants. Consequently there was no other option than to trust Yūsuf and face the mountains.

The journey he planned was well over 200 kilometres and would take us through Podgorica, the capital of Montenegro.

It was a pleasant enough morning. Light snow flurries swept down from time to time but the road was clear of traffic, free from ice and fairly straight. Bernadette and I sat in the back but now Yūsuf stopped for a friend who wanted a ride to Podgorica. We put him between us and, because he was a big fellow, this meant that the three of us were unpleasantly squeezed in the back seat against one another. We had no idea who the friend was but we knew better than to ask too many questions. The main thing was that we were on the way.

In a short time we passed the placid waters of Lake Skadar and proceeded smoothly towards Podgorica, the capital of Montenegro. It was still only eleven o'clock and we were confident that we would reach Peć before dark.

Podgorica was probably the dullest, drabbest and most boring town I have ever been in. The streets were grey, the houses grey and the sky was grey. Traffic was light and no one seemed in a hurry. There was none of the usual city noises of horn hooting or of street vendors haggling their wares that one might expect to find. Instead an air of gloom pervaded the atmosphere and, after stopping for an hour to buy bread and soft drinks, we were happy to get going again. Our passenger left us at this point presumably having hitched a free ride from Yūsuf. We were pleased. It gave us more room in the back.

Initially the countryside was dull and flat although it may have looked more appealing in summer, when the meadows are dotted with wild flowers and the golden harvest sways in the wind. But now, as we left Podgorica, it was a dreary blanket of off-white snow, with just the mountains in the distance to relieve the monotony.

Two hours later, we reached the historic town of Murino, now a mere village, and after that we turned off the main road and faced the mountains and the Čakor Pass which would entail a climb to at least 5000 ft.

Almost at once the road deteriorated and narrowed so that it was impossible for two vehicles to pass each other unless one reversed into a cut-away part of the rock face. The Pass traverses the *Prokletije Planina* range, which roughly translated means the 'Mountains of the Damned' but is more politely named the 'Albanian Alps'. Historically and physically the former is far more apt.

The mountains, which soar to 6000 ft, are criss-crossed with deep canyons and burrowed with caves whose gaping mouths look like puckered black eyes against the snow-encrusted rocks. The hairpin bends were frightening but we drove carefully and, apart from a few small skids on the tarred parts (for some of the road was unpaved), we ascended steadily and actually revelled in the fantastic scenery.

However, our focus was on crossing the border before nightfall and already afternoon mists were rolling down from the mountains. But now we were descending and I think we all breathed a sigh of relief when we saw the border lights loom ahead well before darkness closed in.

Yūsuf was unperturbed. He sped straight on past the line of trucks that were waiting border clearance. 'They risk driving through Čakor but it is worth their while, as they get a bonus for shortening the journey, sometimes by up to 100 d-marks. They save diesel and avoid waiting up to a week at the regular border crossing further north.'

'But is it so dangerous' I interrupted, 'How can they manage to drive those monster trucks up that mountain with the snow and ice?' I might have added 'My God we hardly made it ourselves' but was afraid of insulting Yūsuf's driving skill.

'They will do anything for money. Some of the drivers are from Eritrea … imagine what 100 deutschmarks means to them….' He trailed off. I'm sure it meant a lot to him too.

'They will wait perhaps another day before they get clearance.' It all made sense. I had seen it before.

We stopped right at the barrier and switched on the internal lights as required in many countries, even in daylight. Bernadette and I gave our IDs and passports to Yūsuf, who bade us to stay put. He then got out and went straight to the immigration hut.

He returned in twenty minutes and chuckled 'My cousin is on duty ... no problem.' He started up the engine and proceeded to drive slowly forward. Bernadette was visibly relieved. I am sure she had been as pent up as I all along but did not show it.

We were waved through like royalty. I expect the twenty-dollar bill he suggested I slip into my passport helped expedite matters. He half-turned his head 'We can go straight through ... they wanted to know if you ever met de Valera.'

The three of us laughed and suddenly we all relaxed.

We were through. And it was still light. And yes, he had a cousin on duty there. Thank God for cousins – sometimes.

We now drove rapidly through flat featureless countryside and the land quickly became more inhospitable as dark mountains loomed closer.

Yūsuf was in a talkative mood. He told us all about the Čakor Pass, the White Drin canyon and, the most famed of all, the 25-km long Rugova Canyon, a geological wonder, little known to the outside world. He promised to show us 'the Rugova' on our return journey.

Despite the cold (the car had no heater), despite the tiredness (we had not slept well in Bar) and despite the apprehension that is inevitable when travelling into the unknown, we listened rapt to Yūsuf as he went on and on about the history and geography of the Rugova. And yes, he had guided tourists through this area before the present conflict, a profession he hoped to resume once things got better.

The few short miles to Peć passed quickly thanks to Yūsef's prattle and we hardly felt it before we slowed down on reaching the outskirts of our final destination. Darkness was closing in rapidly.

We made our way slowly through the half-lit streets without incident. Peć rivals Podgorica for being one of the drabbest places I ever saw, but then it is not fair to judge such things in wartime. Indeed Peć boasts many notable buildings including a magnificent Orthodox monastery, now a UNESCO protected site. But that night, as we entered the town, nothing there seemed attractive much less magnificent.

And our lodging was far from magnificent. It was an unpretentious wooden house in an unpretentious street lined by houses which all looked identical. Alicja had rented the place cheaply from a displaced family who were glad of the money. We pulled up in front and gazed in dismay at the shabby and neglected structure. A wave of disappointment passed over me and I could sense that Bernadette felt the same way. 'It'll be grand inside' I assured her. She smiled. Yūsuf fumbled with a bunch of keys and eventually selected the right one. The door opened after he gave it a push and then we entered.

It was dark inside and the cold was piercing. There was no heat and no light and a smell of damp pervaded the atmosphere. We ate our ham sandwiches in silence and drank the last of the tea from Bernadette's flask. The paraffin lamp gave out but a pool of light so that most of the room was in darkness. Long shadows flickered on the walls as the wick waxed and waned. I would not like to have been there on my own. Even Yūsuf was silent. Night fell fast.

Bernadette was given the only bedroom but had to make do on a bare spring base, as there was no mattress. We men lay down on the floor of the living room. We all had sleeping bags but they were inferior things, and none of us took off our coats much less undressed. I will never forget how cold I was that night. I curled myself up in a ball but could not keep warm. In the morning we were like three icicles. Three depressed icicles.

And the next few days did little to raise our spirits. We accomplished nothing and saw nothing and with the usual communication confusion found that the Refugee Trust representative in Peć was missing, nowhere to be found. Our trip was really a failure.

Yūsuf did his best for us by asking around, but his enquiries were in vain. Someone told him that our man had gone up country to see a refugee camp but we were dubious about that. I think he had just done a runner.

We went to the municipal offices and introduced ourselves. They were glad to give us a list of projects that needed help, which we duly took, assuring them that we would consider each carefully but knowing that our mission here was probably finished. We paid three months' rent in advance to the owners of the house that we slept in, and that at least made one family happy. We would close down the operation as soon as possible.

I have few other memories of Peć apart from cold grey streets, deserted except for an occasional person hurrying along, perhaps going home or perhaps doing some errand.

By sheer coincidence, I came across a family that I had befriended in Camp Neptune earlier in the year and who had returned to their native town and re-possessed their home. That was a happy meeting and I can still see the bright faces of the children and smiling face of the mother as they greeted me like an old friend. However the father, the breadwinner, was missing and they had no idea where he might be. I don't know how they could smile.

They introduced me to a lodger, who told me that he had spent over nine months in the attic of a deserted house in Peć, afraid to show his face outside, for fear of the Serbs. He had been an associate of the missing husband and contributed some sort of stability as well as a little money to this family. His story reminded me of that of Anne Frank except that his story had a better ending.

Perhaps the rigours of our trip over the mountains had been worth it after all.

We left early on a Monday morning. We were happy to leave even though we had accomplished so little. By now the three of us had built up a comradeship that made us feel confident in the face of whatever might happen. And the thought to our hotel rooms in Bar beckoned like a homing beam for Bernadette and I.

Our spirits lightened as we left the city. Yūsuf, in particular, was even more talkative than on the outward journey. Like many I met in the Balkans, Yūsuf smoked a lot. We did not object, for the last thing we wanted was any unpleasantness, and, in any event, we were completely in his hands. First we were to see the Rugova Canyon, as Yūsuf had promised.

Rugova Canyon

The Rugova Mountains form a backdrop to Peć and so we accessed them very soon after leaving for home. Snow began to fall more thickly and a harsh wind swept down from the mountains as we neared the famous gorge. Once or twice the car skidded but Yūsuf managed to keep it on the road with surprising skill. Bernadette and I swayed from side to side each time we lurched around corners. The nicest thing was that the car heater now worked. We were warm at last.

Our internal barometres told us that we were climbing higher and higher and, after passing under a succession of tunnels carved out of the side of the mountains, we became aware of a deep canyon on one side. On those occasions, when we looked out the side window, we got a chill of fear from the sight of so many trucks and cars that had skidded off the road and now lay below helplessly.

Yūsuf warmed to his subject as we went along. He informed us that the walls of the Rugova were 1000-metre high and that there was a terrifying plunge for any vehicle that skidded off the road.

'You will drown if you have not broken your neck' he assured us grimly and added 'maybe drowning is the better fate.'

For deep down below, the dreaded Drini River races along, so that even at sub-zero temperatures it is not completely frozen. Waterfalls and streams from caves in the massive rock-face feed the river and make the Rugova canyon one of the most memorable sights and one of the most dangerous winter drives in all Europe.

It must be a glorious drive in summer. The road is wide enough for two trucks to pass each other and the asphalt surface is without potholes.

Today it is safer and crash barriers are placed at strategic sites. And it is just as awe-inspiring.

We arrived in Bar before dusk, glad to be 'home' again. In order to celebrate our last night there, Yūsuf brought us to a fish restaurant south of Bar and close to the Albanian border. Here we treated ourselves to a fine bottle of Italian red wine. The fish was delicious, the wine excellent, the service fast and the conversation easy and relaxed. We bade him say goodbye to Mrs Yūsuf who preferred not to be on the road at night.

It was in its way a memorable night for Bernadette and me.

On returning to our hotel, we bade Yūsuf goodnight and went to our rooms where we slept soundly with the little heaters on all night.

The following day, Yūsuf took us north to the border of Croatia and bade us goodbye. By this time both Bernadette and I had got to like him very much and we were genuinely sorry when waving goodbye. He looked a forlorn figure as the two of us moved away. We would never see him again.

We crossed the border on foot, this time like old-timers. Yūsuf had arranged Mark, who was waiting for us in Dubrovnik, would meet us once we got through Croatian customs and immigration. This time the arrangements worked out perfectly. There was Mark, standing beside the jeep, waving at us like a long lost cousin.

The sea was now on our left-hand side and sparkled brightly in the clear winter sunshine. We felt we were on the first leg of our journey home, back to Ireland. It was a good feeling.

The Roma

We had hardly gone 30 minutes when we spotted smoke on our right-hand side. I asked what was happening and Mark replied deprecatingly that 'The Roma there … dirty place … Smell … Smell'.

That decided me. I would have to see it for myself. 'No good' Mark insisted 'They live dump ... that place dump'.

Nonetheless he reluctantly veered right and down a sloping path pulling up just short of the camp itself. And Mark was right. The camp was located right in the middle of a dump, presumably where all the garbage from Dubrovnik and other towns was deposited. The Roma lived there in smoky clapboard houses and in tarpaulin-covered shacks, reminiscent of the shantytowns I had seen in Africa and India. At least in those places the days were warm and you could cook outside. Here the days were cold, the nights colder and the place was infested with rats. And yes, there was a smell, not only the natural acrid smell from the dump but also the sweet sickly smell of unwashed humanity.

The Roma are universally disliked, distrusted and even feared. They were originally called gypsies because people thought they came from Egypt but now we believe they originated in the Punjab and only came to Europe in the eighth century. They give allegiance to no country and have their own peculiar code of ethics – to which they strictly adhere. Like some other overtly male-dominated societies, behind closed doors, the women rule the roost.

The camp was strewn out on either side of a central path. This path divided the dump in two. But the Roma 'houses' were not laid out in any kind of order. Some were on the side of the path, others were interspersed between piles of rubble and still others seemed to be little more than human burrows in mountains of garbage.

Only I got out. Before my foot touched the ground I was surrounded by a ragged rabble of children all with their hands out and all looking at me with big brown appealing eyes and innocent looking faces. I handed out 'goodies' which they grabbed eagerly and then ran off. I was barely free of them when the adults converged on me – also with hands outstretched. Now there were more strident pleas for money and food. Previous experience had prepared me for this and I had a goodly supply of small denomination notes, which I dispensed liberally. However, as I was dispensing in this lordly fashion, I became conscious of fingers searching my pockets, and I soon realised that everything I had in them was being carried away. This was cleverly organised for they passed on whatever they found from one person to the next, like ants passing crumbs of food from one to the other.

I was even prepared for this and had nothing of importance in my pockets but, far from being annoyed, I could only pity these poor people so scantily clad in the freezing cold of a Balkan winter. I am certain you would feel the same. One woman in particular wore only a torn shimmy dress and she was as thin as a lath. I felt a rotter as I watched her shiver, while I was in my warm Canadian parka, my two sweaters, my thermal underwear and my fine boots. So in a grand gesture I gave her my parka expecting profuse thanks; all I got from her was more whining and more entreaties for money and clothes. This time I brushed her off, perhaps unkindly.

I hope the parka kept her warm. I know I was miserably cold for the next few days until I managed to borrow a coat from a UN worker in Sarajevo.

We left the Roma in sombre mood and retraced our path back to Sarajevo. Once more, we accepted the hospitality of the 'nuns on the hill' and now we really appreciated our warm beds and clean sheets. Each morning we rented a car so that we could visit our programs in the city and on Friday we made a trip to Banja Luka, the capital of the self-styled Republika Srpska.

Here we visited the local hospital to see what was needed and, of course, everything was needed. The list I made filled four foolscap pages and when I returned to Dublin I submitted it to various drug companies.

Banja Luka was very much a Greek Orthodox city, and it was here I first saw shrines in which you lit candles for the living on the bottom shelf (earth) and candles for the dead on the top shelf (Heaven). Perhaps it was the other way around but definitely the living and dead had separate shelves!

I lit candles on both shelves – took no chances of insulting anybody.

It is always a thrill to see the green patchy fields of Ireland as one's plane descends into Dublin Airport. We welcomed the soft rain and gentle winds that made such a contrast to the fierce cold of the Balkans. But we treasured the warmth of the people we had met there and felt happy that we had played a part, however small, in helping them.

It was to be Bernadette's first and only trip overseas. She died of cancer in January 2012, and many a tear was shed as her coffin was lowered into an icy cold grave in Monaghan, her native town. Doreen and I both attended the funeral. Bernadette was truly a lovely person.

Yet no one is irreplaceable. There will always be people like Bernadette willing to work and suffer for others. That is the great hope for mankind.

THE BIAFRAN WAR
1967–1970

Secession of the South

Nigeria became an independent nation on the 1st of October 1960.

Thanks to the work of the British Colonial Administrator Frederick Lugard and his wife Flora one federal state was forged out of three great nations. It was a mongrel state. The new 'Nigeria' was an amalgam of the vast Northern region that was inhabited by the Hausa-Fulani people who were mostly Muslim, the Southwest region inhabited by the Yoruba – mostly Christian, and the Southeast region inhabited by the Igbos, also mostly Christian. In all the three Regions, many still subscribed to traditional religions in their hearts, although they might outwardly be Christian or Muslim.

However in cultural, historical and governance terms each region was completely different, and there was constant bickering between the three. This was most marked in the north where periodic pogroms against the Igbos took place. These culminated in a major persecution in 1966 when thousands of Igbos living in the North were killed. Those who fled told stories of brutalities such as disembowelling, torture and rape, and some say this was the immediate reason for Colornel Ojuka declaring the Republic of Biafra on May 30 1967.

Biafra, the homeland of the Igbos, was the richest and best developed area in the nascent Federal Republic of Nigeria. The similarities between the embryonic Biafra and the now thriving independent state of Israel were not lost on the powers in Lagos, then the Federal capital. Indeed, in common parlance the Igbos were often referred to as the 'Jews of Nigeria'.

The blood and tears of Igbos living in the north had finally awakened the dormant seeds of southern secession. But others believed that oil was the real reason. Shell-BP was the sole concessionaire for the vast oil deposits in the Delta region and once revenues started pouring in from 1958 onwards, everyone wanted a major stake in the new-found wealth.

Britain's interest lay in protecting Shell-BP and so they armed and supported Federal Nigeria in what was legally a civil war, the secession of part of a sovereign state. Ultimately this proved decisive and the 'rebellion' ended officially on 15 January 1970, after almost three years of bloody and merciless fighting.

Special Irish Interest

The Biafran War was the first major conflict and first major famine ever seen on a daily basis as it was actually happening thanks to the miracle of television.

In Ireland people were appalled at the things they saw on their flickering black and white TVs. Most had a relative or knew someone who was a missionary in Nigeria and so there was also a strong emotional tie between the Irish and the Igbos.

For Irish Republicans, it was the association of southern Nigeria – *le bas Niger* – with the tragic Roger Casement that meant most. For Catholics the names Calabar, the Bight of Biafra and Port Harcourt evoked memories of Bishop Shanahan of the Holy Ghost Fathers (nowadays the 'Spiritans'), and for Protestants it was the image of Mary Slessor, the intrepid young Scottish girl who went to Calabar in the late 1800s to 'convert the heathen'.

For me there was a fourth link that was strongest of all. And that was Mary Martin, the young Dublin woman who had founded the Medical Missionaries of Mary, the MMMs. She had started her African mission among the Igbos in 1937 when I was three years old. Her aim was to serve the sick and her special emphasis was on serving women and children who were the most neglected of all. She had nothing but hope, determination and an indomitable optimism well expressed in the MMM motto 'rooted in love'.

Her first hospital in Africa was in a place called Anua, and she named it St Lukes.

I was born on St Luke's day and so I felt it a good omen when the International Committee of the Red Cross (the ICRC) sent me to St Luke's hospital in Anua.

Year of Hope and Hopelessness

It was 1969, the year when Neil Armstrong and Buzz Aldrin became the first men to land on the moon, a year that is remembered by most for the cleverness and bravery of mankind.

Instead I remember it as the year when the Biafran War was reaching its climax, when hundreds of thousands of

Nigerians were made homeless and when over two million innocent people were either killed or deliberately starved to death.

Yet it was also a year when the goodness of mankind shone through. People all over the world raised money for the relief of the suffering they saw before their eyes. Numerous new governmental and NGOs sprang up to give direct aid. There was an outpouring of generosity on an unprecedented scale.

Among the most significant NGOs started in Ireland was Africa Concern, founded in 1968. It was the time too when USAID, OXFAM CAFOD, CRS (Catholic Relief Services) and individual Red Cross Societies came of age and played crucial roles in providing people with food and shelter and medical supplies. And it was the time that gave birth to MSF.

Médecins Sans Frontières

Médecins Sans Frontières (MSF) was officially founded in 1971 mainly due to the reaction of two French doctors, Max Recamier and Bernard Kouchner, to their experiences in Biafra. During that time, they became disillusioned with the ICRC (International Committee of the Red Cross) for its policy of standing aside from political issues – irrespective of who was right and who was wrong – and for refraining to condemn those who obviously promoted evil. They reckoned the ICRC was too 'neutral' and was imposing a gag order on its workers, which precluded them from speaking the truth.

The ICRC felt justified because otherwise it would certainly be stopped from helping those most in need and would be seen as favouring one side over the other.

Whatever views you have, it is clear that the ICRC and MSF complement each other and that both are needed. They are two sides of the same coin.

Conflict of Interests

But as you can imagine, this sudden rush to help was dysfunctional and un-coordinated. Groups frequently duplicated services and money was wasted. Aid groups were often ill-prepared and un-professional, and some-times disputed acrimoniously with one another for control of the same patch of territory.

As a result, much time, money and effort were wasted despite the best intentions of all concerned. Nor should we forget that corruption and bureaucratic obstacles in the receiving country compounded the problem. The wonder is that any meaningful aid got through at all. One example illustrates this well. Gorta, an Irish aid organisa-tion, had raised over £100,000 to send supplies to Nige-ria. To do this, they sent several ships all loaded with humanitarian supplies destined for those in greatest need. I suspect they were quite shocked to find that they could only discharge their cargoes in Lagos if a large sum of money was paid in excise duties. But look at the matter from the point of view of the Federal Government of Nige-ria (FGN). They saw themselves trying to crush a rebellion and here was the West sending relief to their enemies, relief that would surely go first to those actively fighting against them. Furthermore, it was the stated policy of the FGN to starve the 'Biafrans' into submission. To many Nigerians, this was arrogant interference in an internal matter.

São Tomé

It was quickly realised that the only way to get aid to the starving Igbos was to bypass Federal territory. The obvious route was to channel it through São Tomé, a small friendly Portuguese island in the Bight of Biafra. Initially Africa Concern sent the 600-ton MV Columcille loaded with supplies to São Tomé and soon the island became a two-way staging post, bringing aid into and carrying people out of the beleaguered enclave. The Irish public eventually contributed over £3.5 million to Africa Concern, much of it spent in sending relief ships.

Later air transport became even more important. It was started at the behest of the Catholic and Protestant Churches who were appalled at reports of 1,000 children dying of starvation every day. The Biafran airlift, between Biafra and São Tomé, ultimately became the largest such operation since the Berlin airlift of the Cold War days.

U Thant, the Secretary General of the UN, refused to support the airlift and failed to condemn outrightly the FGN when it imposed a total blockade on Biafra in 1968. Nor did anyone seriously challenge the FGN spokesman who declared in 1968 that 'starvation is a legitimate weapon of war ... and we have every intention of using it against the rebels.'

Some say the use of São Tomé prolonged the war; others argue that it saved many lives. Probably it did both.

For my part all I felt able to do was help on a person-to-person, a one-to-one basis. In later life, I realised that I could have made a better, more lasting and more important contribution, had I been more political in nature and spent more time in administration, in making political contacts and in garnering widespread support for the concepts of peace and justice.

People such as Christine Noble on the one hand and Bob Geldof on the other have made far more significant contributions to alleviating suffering than I, precisely because they made people and governments move from their natural lethargy. And yet, if each one contributes just a little, whether money, time or skill, according to his or her capabilities, then world would surely change beyond recognition.

APPENDIX 2

WITCH DOCTORS

Very Special People

Witch doctors were an important, respected and often feared part of society in 'my' Africa. They did far more than treat physical disease in the local population. They placated the spirits on behalf of their suppliants, they helped control the weather, they resolved family and tribal issues, they brought good luck on those who paid them obeisance and, more importantly, they could bring bad luck down on one's enemies. They also predicted the future – sometimes with uncanny accuracy. All these things the witch doctor did using small animals, snakes and other symbols to communicate their wishes to some higher power and in doing so they sometimes went into a trance like a state similar to the shamans of Asia.

Witch doctors were specially chosen either on family grounds or by selection from a group of pre-pubertal boys who were subject to examination and scrutiny by the elders of the community.

Some years ago, one of my students, while doing an elective in Kenya, recorded on film a very special ritual for choosing a new medicine man or witch doctor, whatever you may wish to call him. The event took place in a small village on the banks of Lake Victoria, some miles north of the town of Kisumu.

It was dusk, the short dusk of the tropics, when a group of six young boys were stripped of their clothes and brought naked down to the shores of the lake by a large group of male villagers. The pictures show these boys, firmly held, and looking scared. All had curiously dilated pupils as if they had been given some atropine-like drug. By the time they reached the lakeshore it was dark, but there was enough light from a bright moon to clearly illuminate the scene. At this point one boy alone was selected. I do not know why they selected this boy but clearly it was a pre-arranged choice. There was no arguing, no protests from anyone, no noise save the rustling of the trees and the lapping of the lake water. The boy's hands were now firmly bound with white cotton bandages and the men then proceeded to cover him completely with soft mud scooped up from the lakeshore or should I say seashore, for Lake Victoria resembles more a sea than a lake and, in truth, that is what it is, since it is tidal and subject to terrible storms.

It was on the banks of this great lake, a lake that seems to me to be the epicentre of all the lakes in the world, that the next piece of the drama unfolded. Several men surrounded the chosen boy and, judging by the child's screams, they must have hurt him and hurt him a lot despite all their incantations and potions. Suddenly the screams became a whimper and he was set free.

Set free as a eunuch for life. But a special eunuch. A witch doctor. The village advisor, healer, prophet and sorcerer. A man to be feared and respected. A person who would be treated from that moment on with special reverence. He will not have to work; the villagers will provide for his every need, and beware the person who dares cross him in any way.

Scarification

Tribal scarification is common in Africa, many tribes having specific patterns by which they can be identified. There are many reasons for painting, etching and scarifying the skin. Apart from conferring a definable social status, the reasons vary from aesthetic and cultural to a power that enables the person to be healed both in mind and body.

The actual scarification process is usually accompanied by dancing, the wearing of masks, rhythmic music, drum beating and the consumption of large amount of local beer. All this helps put the whole company into a state of euphoria and helps remove the element of pain from the proceedings.

In cases of sickness, the witch doctor may be called on to scarify the offending part. I have seen the value of this when cuts were made deep enough to let pus drain from an underlying abscess. Unfortunately, more often than not, scarification is either of no use or harmful. Thus patients with abdominal pain, say from a volvulus (twisted intestines), might have their abdominal skin raked with knives, or their back may be scarified in cases of backache. I have seen this in cases of Pott's disease (TB of the spine).

Scarifying little children frequently allows infection to spread and may result in a life-threatening septicaemia (blood poisoning) and in many cases large ugly thickening of the scarified edges occurs, which we call keloids – ugly, disfiguring lumps of overgrown scar tissue.

The Evil One

In Igboland, the witch doctor was called a dibia or juju man, and it was believed that many dibias had direct connections with the Evil One, Ekwensu, or Satan – as we might say. Sometimes whole villages were totally under the thrall of a dibia who plunged it into every kind of vice imaginable.

Old missionary tales recount the unseen presence of a force physically preventing the missioner from entering such cesspools of evil. Bishop Shanahan writes graphically about his experiences in this regard, so graphically that one feels he truly grappled with something dark and inexplicable at times.

This 'bad' kind of dibia ordered the slaughter of babies and the ritual murder of children in an effort to maintain his power and status in his village. He would explain that this was necessary in order to placate the spirits. Otherwise great misfortune would follow. Sometimes, when asked a special favour, the dibia would slaughter an animal, but if this failed, and as a last resort, he would resort to human sacrifice.

Human sacrifice was an honour unless the victim was judged to be the cause of some bad luck such as crop failure or death of a loved one. Strangers were the usual victims. Indeed – even if the dibia did not command it – the norm was to kill any stranger who approached a village.

Human sacrifice reached a zenith in 1918 when the land was swept by the great influenza pandemic and people turned in desperation to the dibia for help. When people recovered, the dibia was fêted. When someone died, the dibia joined in the mourning, but pointed out that the person's death was necessary in order to prevent a greater tragedy occurring. Although it was clearly against the law, human sacrifice continued sporadically for many years afterwards.

No wonder we spoke in hushed tones whenever we talked about the strange happenings on JuJu Hill which was quite near Mile 4 Hospital where I worked.

Master-Spirits

The two master-spirits that govern all things, according to long established beliefs in southern Nigeria, are Cukwu (Good) and Ekwensu (Evil).

These are regarded as too aloof and too busy with celestial affairs to concern themselves with everyday life on earth. They delegate this work to lesser spirits who are good or evil, compassionate or spiteful depending on which master-spirit they represent.

Cukwu and Ekwensu are also regarded as too sublime for humans to worship directly, so all sacrifices and offerings are made through their subordinates. This parallels 'intermediaries' in many religions such as 'saints' in Christianity. Even in the most remote areas no one believed that any work of man, such as statues, amulets or charms, had intrinsic power. Nor did anyone believe that animate or inanimate manifestations of nature had any special power.

However, they did believe that Cukwu or Ekwensu often infused lesser spirits into such things and that the dibia, and only the dibia, had the power to mollify or displease these lesser spirits. He did this, on behalf of the people, by using special chants and invocations and dances – all of which modern man dismisses as mumbo-jumbo. Yet many of the pagan rituals closely resembled those practised by the major religions of the Western World. And this facilitated rather than hindered the spread of Christianity, and to a lesser extent of Islam, in pagan lands.

Second Burial

One of the most fascinating roles of the dibia was to preside at a second burial. Pagans in southern Nigeria always had two burials.

The first burial consisted of burying the body. This was similar to burial in the West, except that the grieving was far more demonstrative, especially on the part of the women. After the first burial some women grieved so excessively that they actually killed themselves or ended up mentally deranged for life. Only the intervention of other women could prevent such a double tragedy.

The more important second burial took place several weeks later. This was a celebration, in which the bereaved consigned the spirit of the dead person into the arms of Chukwu, and the more flamboyantly they did it the greater their hope that the dead person's spirit would be grateful and in turn protect them.

Respect for Paganism

Clearly the pagans of southern Nigeria believe – and believe strongly – in an afterlife, and in a vibrant communion between the living and the dead. Clearly, they also believe that human artefacts and natural phenomena can be used as instruments to propitiate Chukwu or ward off Ekwensu. That is, they believe in Good and Evil. And clearly, they believe in the precedence of the spirit over the body. And this philosophy was not confined to the Igbos. For example, the Baganda of Central Africa also believe in Good (Katonda) and Evil (many names). Surely, an analogy to the Judaeo-Christian Yahweh and Lucifer strikes one forcibly.

Although the pantheon of the Yoruba in western Nigeria consists of no less than 400 gods, it still holds to one supreme creator, called Oluron. He is too much above us to be represented by any statue and even too much above us to be worshipped. It is interesting – and comforting for the Yoruba – to know that they have no real evil Satan. The nearest they have is Ogun who takes fun in trying us. A trickster god.

Because of these analogies, some equate the dibia – the witch doctor – with rabbis, priests, pastors, imans, mullahs. I think this is rather pushing things too far!

Nonetheless surely we should recognise that paganism is not all mumbo jumbo. Much in paganism promotes honesty, fidelity and self-control for a higher purpose.

Overall the art of the witch doctor was aimed at healing illness, bringing rain, ensuring a good harvest, or a good marriage, and in generally benefiting his village. Whatever the blanket of mumbo-jumbo ritual they used, it is clear that the dibia was held in respect – often in dread – by those around him.

However, there was one thing that the dibia himself feared, and that was losing face. In this respect, he differed little from modern medical doctors.

Traditional Medicines

Many of our modern medicines derive from those used in the past by witch doctors and traditional healers. For example, the modern cure for malaria is directly based on the ancient Chinese practise of giving an extract of the common herb *Artemisia annua* for 'fever'. And before the West embraced the 'artemisinins', it relied heavily on Jesuit's bark (quinine), another traditional plant product, this time used in South America. In India psychoses and high blood pressure were treated with an extract of Indian snakeroot, which is the basis for several of today's drugs for these conditions.

And most people have heard of the cardiac effects of foxglove (digitalis) discovered by Europeans in the late 1700s. Native tribes have used foxglove for 'dropsy' (heart failure) from time immemorial.

Extracts of plants containing curare or belladonna have been used by traditional healers for centuries and nowadays play an important role in medical treatment. However, most of us know of them from reading crime thrillers where they are regularly used as a way to murder someone.

Finally – in my own experience – I have seen a witch doctor giving an extract of special roots to procure an abortion. Scientific analysis proved that the extract could do just that.

APPENDIX 3

UGANDA: THE PEARL OF AFRICA

The story of Uganda is a long, sad and bloody one. Much has been lost in the mists of time, much of what has been handed down is distorted, more like mythology than history, but much has also been preserved, in particular stories about the Buganda nation, the largest and most important kingdom in Uganda.

The inhabitants of Buganda are ethnic Bantus, and are called Baganda or Ganda. They are fine-looking people, with a proud fearless bearing complemented with a striking inborn courtesy. As a group they thrived – without outside interference – for many centuries, and developed a religion and culture and a way of life that was as distinctive and rich as could be found anywhere in the world. Laws were codified and strictly enforced, and were all ultimately based on obedience to a primary *Creator* which they called Katonda.

Nonetheless Baganda monotheism differed fundamentally from the great monotheistic religions in that it was believed that Katonda ruled via a series of secondary gods, all of whom were accessible to prayer and sacrifice. As a result, there were many holy places where livestock such as cows and goats were sacrificed. On special occasions, human sacrifice was practised but we have no record of how often this occurred.

Bagandans have told me stories of man's origin which are very similar to the biblical one of Adam and Eve. Instead of Adam, they called the first man Kintu, and this was a name so revered that the first recorded Kabaka (king) of Buganda, Kato Kintu, took it for himself. They also believed that mankind was redeemed in some mysterious way and there are many different versions of their redemption story.

Over many centuries the lives of the ordinary Baganda were governed harshly. Morality was rigidly imposed, on pain of terrible consequences, including torture and beheading.

However, by the sixteenth century, the gods of the Sesse islanders, from Lake Victoria, gradually replaced the traditional Baganda ones. The new religion eschewed the strict morality of the ancient one and gradually replaced it by idolatry, witchcraft, sorcery and many heinous practises.

Despite this change, society remained strictly authoritarian. Deference to those of higher social standing became even more dominant and people's daily lives were ruled in almost every detail by decrees from those above them. Sometimes these decrees were sensible, but mostly they were whimsical at best and outrageous at worst.

The chain of authority was strictly hierarchical. The Kabaka was at the top. He, and he alone, embodied supreme power and had unquestioned control over the life and death of all his subjects.

Our history, therefore, is inextricably bound with that of the Kabakas, the kings of Buganda.

The Kabakas

By the fourteenth century Buganda was a coherent and powerful state. From that time on a series of despotic

Kabakas ruled unchallenged until 1966 when Milton Obote abolished their kingdom in a decisive effort to create a unified single state called Uganda.

The first Kabaka, Katu Kintu, had set the lifestyle for his successors. It was a life of splendour. He was constantly surrounded by vassal lieges and by obedient women and pageboys. These acceded to his every wish no matter how bizarre and outrageous it might be.

In theory, the palace drums (Mujaguzo drums) were actually more important than the Kabaka. They were regarded as sacred and embodied the wishes of the gods. When sounded, everyone had to obey their command.

In practise there was a simple way for the Kabaka to exert his authority whenever he wished.

Of course, the drums also played a significant role in palace protocol and were always sounded on the birth of the Kabaka's children and during the accession ceremony for a new Kabaka. But these were merely ceremonial shows, much as the Changing of the Guard outside Buckingham Palace or the sentries at Napoleons tomb in Paris or the Swiss Guards in the Vatican or the ceremonial Guards of Honour in Washington are today.

When Milton Obote's army attacked and ransacked the palace in 1966, in what became known as the battle of Mengo Hill, the soldiers destroyed the sacred drums. This sad desecration symbolised the beginning of the end of the long reign of the Kabakas. Obote, who led Uganda to independence from Britain in 1962, was from northern Uganda, and had no love for Buganda much less for its 'king'.

King Freddie

The final death knell to the reign of the Kabakas was sounded by the exile and death of King 'Freddie', Mutesa 11, the last true Kabaka of Buganda in 1969.

The British had first wooed Mutesa 11. He was educated in Britain and took a degree in Cambridge and had even become a captain in the Grenadier Guards. All this was done to make him look favourably on Britain. But when he came to power, instead of being a pawn of the British, he went his own way, so much so that the British forcibly exiled him a few years after his homecoming.

His deportation from Kampala was both audacious and ignominious. The unfortunate man was driven in broad daylight to Entebbe airport, with a blanket covering his head, as if he were a common criminal.

This shocked ordinary Ugandans who kept up pressure on the United Kingdom for his return. London relented and reinstated him. But sadly his efforts to re-assert his power as king of an independent Buganda came to nothing.

Britain looked on sceptically. A strong united Uganda was not really in their interest whereas a looser multi-tribal state was, and this coincided with the wishes of Milton Obote. And so they decided to exile him a second time.

The second exile was worse than the first. This time Mutesa 11 fled Uganda in degrading and dangerous circumstances and was forced to smuggle himself into neighbouring Burundi. Here he appealed for sanctuary and was lucky to have friends there who pitied him. From aspiring to rule a great and progressive kingdom he was now a penniless beggar.

And then an unexpected piece of good fortune came his way. Britain repented its handling of the whole affair and allowed him come to live in the United Kingdom where he was received with dignity and courtesy.

And yet, understandably, he longed for home. His wishes were unfulfilled and he died in exile in London in 1969. Many believe he was poisoned.

The western press headlined the death of 'King Freddie'. I never liked that name. For me it cheapens the title Kabaka, and belittles a dynasty that ruled a great kingdom for longer than most European nations were in existence.

A Pathetic Compromise

Perhaps it was conscience, perhaps it was expediency, but whatever the reason, President Museveni invited King Freddie's son Ronald Muwenda II back to Uganda in 1993, and restored a sham monarchy. The people cheered and fêted the return of their Kabaka and the world applauded Museveni's benevolence.

But the Kabaka today has no political power, no real standing. He functions as a tawdry enfeebled version of the Kabakas of old.

On my last visit to his present abode, I found that persons 'unknown' had burned it down, and all that remained was a few scattered thatch roofed huts which were visited by the occasional tourist, and which were minded by a handful of indifferent caretakers.

Come the Colonists and the Clerics

Speke and Grant arrived in the Kingdom of Buganda in January 1862. They were the first Europeans to do so. It was Speke's third trip to Central Africa, having previously gone to Somaliland in 1852 to collect botanical specimens and four years later with Richard Burton in a fruitless search for the source of the Nile.

These Victorian explorers came with the hope of ultimately exploiting the vast riches of central Africa. But in fairness, they did not come to engage in the thriving slave trade, which was predominantly in the hands of unscrupulous Arabs. However – to their shame – they did co-operate with the slave trade when it suited their purposes.

Livingstone spoke of slavery as 'the open sore of the world'. But words are only words and, although Wilberforce had unambiguously condemned slavery in the House of Commons as early as 1792, it was not abolished in reality until well into the nineteenth century.

The truth is that, while the Victorian explorers did little to eradicate slavery, they did make the world more aware of the practice, and in so doing, they undoubtedly reinforced moves by the Christian churches to establish missions, in which everyone was safe and free.

Missionaries, Mercenaries and Merchants

We may admire their courage but it is difficult to like the Victorian explorers.

They all seemed to crave fame and in pursuit of this were extremely jealous of one another and openly traded mutual insults. Many were prepared to deal with the slave traders in order to further their aims, despite pretending to stand for Christian principles. Others, for example Stanley, were indifferent to the suffering of the natives and actually seemed to enjoy murdering them in cold blood. Even David Livingstone – often hailed as a living saint in

England – imposed hardships on his native servants that were unfair and inhumane.

Viewed by today's standards, it is difficult to see how the explorers could believe they treated their workers reasonably. Perhaps we should be kinder to them were we to judge them by the standards of the late 1800s and not by our own.

In 1862, on their first meeting, Mutesa 1st, the Kabaka, had welcomed Speke warmly and Speke felt the meeting was a great success. Privately Speke declared he was aghast at 'the tales of human sacrifice ... torture and execution for the most trivial offenses ... even for speaking too loudly in the king's presence.' Yet to the Kabaka's face he was most agreeable, probably because he feared for his own safety.

However, the Kabaka's benevolent reception had altered completely by February 1879 when Speke and Grant sailed across Lake Victoria and landed in Entebbe. Then they were humiliated and finally completely ignored.

This was neither bad manners nor a lack of hospitality on the part of the Kabaka. He was actually playing off the Catholics against the Protestants and would later include the Muslims in his political carousel, all the time looking for the best deal he could get.

Eventually he did grant them an audience and accepted their mission to Buganda. Yet he diplomatically left them in no doubt that they were there only at his pleasure.

Protestant Missionaries

The first Christian missionaries to Uganda were Anglicans and were spearheaded by Lt. Shergold Smith and the Rev

C. T. Wilson of the Church Missionary Society (CMS). They came in June 1877, two years before the Catholics.

They set up in Mengo Hill, close to the residence of the Kabaka, and were not only committed Christians but were also brave and fearless men. Smith was killed in December less than six months after his arrival, and so Wilson was left on his own. Poor Wilson was beset with illness, isolation and loneliness for the next year.

It was then that a most able and zealous compatriot, Alexander Mackay, a young Scottish engineer, joined him. Mackay arrived in Uganda in November 1878 and worked tirelessly to promote not just his brand of Christianity but also to establish schools, medical clinics and trades.

His constant work earned him the name Mzungwa Kazi (white man work) but inevitably he died of malaria before he was 50 years old.

Catholic Missionaries

Thomas Packenham in *The Scramble for Africa* entitles one chapter 'The Flag follows the Cross'. And this is certainly true of Uganda. The first Catholic missionaries to go there were Fr Simeon Lourdel and his companion Brother Amans. These belonged to a new French Missionary Society that had been founded in 1868 by Charles Lavigerie, the Archbishop of Algiers, then a French colony. Members were known as 'The White Fathers' – not because most were fair skinned, but because of their long white Arab cassocks and red fezzes.

Their founder was one of the most remarkable clerics of the age and more than earned his unofficial title of 'Cardinal of Africa'. His stance on slavery was clear, unequivocal and passionate: he denounced the practise eloquently and continually in writings and speeches all his life.

After his death in 1892, the numbers of White Fathers increased until by 1950 there were 2500 'White Fathers' and as many Sisters and lay people working in Africa.

Catholic Protestant Rivalry

Unfortunately the rivalry that existed between Catholics and Protestants in Europe continued in Uganda. This sullied the reputation of both groups and was exploited by the Kabakas who sat back and played one group against the other, all the time extracting the maximum advantage for themselves and secretly enjoying the overt hostility that existed between the two 'brands' of Christianity.

Meanwhile, in the secular sphere, the English and French were vying for political influence, but neither seemed credible in view of the identification of each with specific and antagonistic religions; England with Protestantism and France with Catholicism.

In 1894 the English made the first concrete move to address this. In that year they encouraged Bishop Léon Livinhac, one of the French White Fathers in Uganda, to invite the Mill Hill fathers from Britain to join them. It was an astute move and one that showed clearly to the Kabaka that not all English were Protestant.

At that particular moment, the Kabaka wanted to curry favour from the French Catholics and so was delighted when the Protestant English sent seven Mill Hill missionaries to Kampala. They were warmly welcomed by an apparently friendly Kabaka when they arrived in September 1895. He even gave them a gift of Nsambya Hill in Kampala – the site of the future St Francis hospital where

I would work 78 years later. Unfortunately time would reveal that this benevolence was more apparent than real.

Missionaries and Slavery

Apart from condemning slavery from their pulpits, the Christian missionaries, both Catholic and Protestant, tried hard to put their aspirations into practise. An example of this was the work of the Holy Ghost Fathers in their mission near the coastal town of Bagamoyo, the original capital of German East Africa, now Tanzania.

This mission was specifically located to free and house Africans from the slave gangs that passed that way. The priests paid over the odds especially for weak and elderly slaves. The slave masters were glad to get rid of these for they who would bring little money on the open market. Indeed they must have rubbed their hands with glee as they pocketed their Judas money. For now, they could press on to Zanzibar unencumbered by less desirable slaves and save money on food to boot.

Once in Zanzibar, the unfortunates who had not been freed would be chained up in holding pens. There they would die or be sold and shipped overseas like cattle.

The stories of what happened in those days are still told in Zanzibar where today's visitor can see the original holding pens and slave markets. It is difficult to comprehend how men could have treated other human beings in such a fashion.

The Great Hospitals of Kampala

These exist today as important legacies of the early Christian missionaries.

St Francis Catholic hospital, on Nsambya Hill, was founded in 1903 by Mother Kevin or Mama Kevin, as she was affectionately known. Mama Kevin, born Teresa Kearney in 1875 in Co. Wicklow, was a truly remarkable woman. She was energetic, far seeing, lovable – and holy. She arrived in Uganda in 1903 as a member of the Franciscan Missionary Sisters for Africa and served that country faithfully all her working life.

Nsambya hospital traces its origin to a small bush clinic that Mother Kevin's sisters started under a mango tree in 1903. From this small beginning has arisen the busy modern hospital that I last visited in 2014. I do not think that in her wildest dreams Mama Kevin would have imagined that such a legacy was possible. But her delight would be doubled to see that it is now in the hands of African Sisters, the Little Sisters of St Francis, and is fully integrated into Uganda's medical service. Yet it was not in Nsambya that her body was buried on 3rd December 1957 but 50 km southeast of Kampala in Nkokonjeru. This was by popular demand of the people of Nkokonjeru who had their beloved Mama brought back from Boston where she had died.

Nkokonjeru had been the scene of one of her greatest triumphs. It was here she vanquished the local Baganda god, the White Cock.

There was a sacred tree in Nkokonjeru on which it was alleged that an evil spirit, in the form of a white cock, perched from time to time and would bring disaster on anyone who failed to make sacrifices to it. The tree was taboo to the locals. But not to Mama Kevin. One evening it was struck by lightning and toppled to the ground. Mama Kevin saw this as a gift sent from heaven to be used in the construction of a local church and convent. She started sawing the tree into handy-sized logs.

No one dared help her. People stared in awe, expecting evil spirits to burn her up, but instead she worked away unharmed. One by one they joined her. This earned the white-robed Mama Kevin another sobriquet, 'The White Hen'.

Which was fitting; the White Hen had got the better of the White Cock!

The great Protestant hospital, Mengo Hospital, was built on Namirembe Hill and is the oldest hospital in East Africa. An outstanding Englishman, Sir Albert Cook, founded it in 1897. Albert Cook was a dedicated CMS missionary who worked selflessly for the people of Uganda and for the furtherance of medicine in that country.

His brother, a surgeon, joined him in his work, and Katherine, a missionary nurse whom he married in 1900, helped him found a School of Nursing. A nephew, Ernest Cook, joined the group in 1907 and brought the first X-ray machine to East Africa. For the Cooks it was almost a 'family affair'.

Not far from Mengo Hospital you come across the lovely Anglican cathedral of St Paul. It was appropriate that the Anglicans chose to build their place of spiritual healing near their place of physical healing.

However, Albert Cook was not content with founding just one hospital. He was also largely responsible for founding a second one. This happened in 1913 and the site was yet another of Kampala's hills, this time Mulago Hill. Mulago, with almost 2000 beds, is now the national referral hospital for Uganda and is the teaching hospital for the nearby University of Makerere, one of the most important centres of learning and academic excellence in Africa.

In 1951, Albert Ruskin Cook, one of the great benefactors of Uganda, died at the age of 81 in his beloved

Kampala – coincidentally the year I started my medical studies in UCD.

Islam's Turn

Islam first came to Uganda in 1844 with the advent of Arab slave traders. It was the first major outside religion to arrive. The fact that it condoned polygamy suited the local way of living and gave it a head start over strictly monogamous Christianity.

Furthermore, the Kabaka at the time, Mutese 1st, strongly espoused it. He – and his advisors – did so because the slave trade filled their coffers. But slavery was hated and feared by the masses for whom it brought nothing but misery and degradation. So most people turned to Christianity – especially to Roman Catholicism – where the use of emblems, amulets, statues and other sacramentals fitted seamlessly into their traditional rituals.

Many combined Christianity, Islam and Paganism by publicly professing Christianity, privately keeping many wives, and secretly deferring to ancient rituals and taboos.

Muslims have always exerted a political significance far beyond their numbers and several Kabakas of Buganda and Presidents of Uganda have been born Muslim or changed to that faith. Indeed, a visit to Kampala today is not complete without going to the National Mosque, a gift from Muammar Gaddafi of Libya. It is a stunning building atop Kampala Hill and a sign of the power of Islam which offers certainty in an uncertain world.

Although nominally a Muslim, Mutesa 1st made temporary alliances with whatever religion suited his purposes best. Hence he lost no time in inviting Christian missionaries – English Protestant and French Catholic – to his country. He then sat back and watched the fun.

Mutesa 1st and Mwanga 2nd

Into this mix, of Catholics, Protestants, Muslims and Native Religions, was thrown the political rivalry between England and France and, to a lesser extent, Germany. No wonder the pragmatic, sometimes cunning, and often barbaric Kabaka Mutesa 1st must have enjoyed watching the foreigners squabble among themselves. Mutesa 1st was in fact the 31st Kabaka and held office until his death in 1884.

Sometimes he favoured one side, then the other, as his whims dictated. But always he expected to gain something in return. His son and successor Mwanga 2nd succeeded him in 1884.

Mwanga 2nd was an even more brutal, despotic and Hitler-like tyrant. He changed his religion to suit his pocket but in his heart he particularly hated the Christians.

This hatred was fanned into flames when the Christians denounced as 'unnatural' many of the practises he engaged in, especially that of having sex with his pageboys. We shall see that he had his revenge on the Christians, a revenge that was to prove short-lived and ultimately provoke the outrage of the civilised world.

Fredrick Lugard 1890–1992

As far as political acumen was concerned, Mwanga 2nd met his match in Captain Frederick Lugard DSO, the young representative of the Imperial British East Africa

Company (IBEAC) and a British military administrator of outstanding ability.

Lugard's personal history, as a dashing soldier in India, of unrequited love and of his final happy marriage to Flora, reads like a novel. Yet he had a constancy of purpose that belied his capricious youth. His life purpose in Uganda was simple. It was to incorporate the whole of Uganda into the British Empire.

To do so, he needed to pacify Buganda and, as part of this, he tried to make common cause with other Europeans so that they would act together as a united force and respect each other's religion.

He had first-hand knowledge of how Britain behaved in India where she acted as a central power bestowing land and privileges on local potentates and backing only those who were clearly friendly to the Crown. Now he planned to do the same thing in Uganda. The gain for England would be control over the riches of the whole region. The gain for Uganda would be a Pax Britannica. The gain for Lugard would be recognition as the man who inserted another jewel into the crown of the British monarch.

Mwanga thought long and hard and came to the conclusion that going along with Lugard was probably the best thing to do. One of the things that swayed him in favour of England – as against Germany, Egypt or France – was Lugard's policy of non-interference with the practises of local rulers. Mwanga and his henchmen could continue to indulge themselves as much as ever and still maintain their prestige among the people.

Yet we can detect a note of regret too when Mwanga wrote:

'They (the English) have come ...they have eaten my land ... they have given me nothing at all.'

This they did.

Lugard moved on to the West Coast once he had accomplished his mission in Uganda. Indeed his lasting claim to fame is mostly based on the unification of Nigeria into one colony. Flora, his wife, ably assisted him in this, and together they made a formidable team during his term as Governor General of that country (1914–1919).

Namungongo, 1885–1887

Given Lugard's policy of non-interference in local affairs, Mwanga 2nd continued to indulge himself without shame or reserve. In particular, his dislike of Christianity grew steadily. The refusal of several of his pageboys to accede to his sexual demands – Mwanga was a bisexual – particularly irritated him. And so, ignoring international condemnation, he embarked on several anti-Christian pogroms in which he forced Christians to abandon their faith on pain of torture and death. Those who resisted paid the price in full. His irritation was fanned into an obsessional fury when he was told that many were still converting to Christianity. The pogroms became more vicious and more frequent.

All this time IBEAC – the unofficial arm of the British Crown – was powerless to intervene as it deemed religious persecution an internal matter, under the sole jurisdiction of the Kabaka.

However, when Mwanga started expelling foreign missioners, only stopping short of openly murdering them, IBEAC protested strongly. He ignored these protests, knowing well that IBEAC's operations in Uganda depended on his good will.

Seeing that IBEAC was powerless, Mwanga finally decided to make a public example of prominent Christians. By so doing he was sure he could frighten all Christians into accepting his absolute spiritual authority.

And so, in 1885, the deadly lot fell to the unfortunate Sussex born Anglican Archbishop, James Hannington.

The 38-year-old archbishop had approached Uganda from near Mombasa (Kenya) heedless, or perhaps not knowing, of the oracle that predicted Buganda would be conquered from the east. This prediction had upset Mwanga and was, for him, a sufficient political excuse for imprisoning and spearing Hannington and his party within days of their arrival in Buganda. It is likely that the Arab slavers applauded this act since Hannington was a dedicated and outspoken abolitionist.

I do not know why Hannington chose to ignore the warnings from Alexander Mackay, not to take that route. Mackey, a devout Scottish Presbyterian missionary and a clever engineer, was well familiar with the Kabaka's court at this stage, whereas Hannington was a newcomer. It seems that Hanningon was simply a saintly naïve person and probably just trusted that God would mind him.

The Martyrs of Namungongo

Joseph Mukasa was the Majordomo at the Court and was a known convert to Catholicism. He was very popular among the Chiefs because of his pleasant manner, his fair dealing with everyone and because of the way he helped those in trouble.

Outraged at what had happened to Bishop Hannington he foolishly rebuked Mwanga for the murder. He also chided him more foolishly – no – more courageously, for his sexual abuse of the palace pageboys. Joseph probably expected that being the senior official of the Royal Court, he would be immune from serious punishment.

He was quickly disabused of this notion. Within days he was arrested and, on 15th November 1885, he was summarily beheaded. This was at the instigation of the Katikkiro (Prime Minister) and some older chiefs who feared that power would pass to the popular Majordomo.

For once Anglicans and Roman Catholics, not only in Uganda, but everywhere, were united in their shocked reaction. But this only made matters worse. For the next two years all Christians of whatever denomination were fair game and were hunted ruthlessly, and anyone who resisted was martyred.

The culmination of the massacres occurred when 24 young Roman Catholics and 21 young Anglicans, all mere boys, were burned alive because they would not renounce their Christianity and would not accede to Mangwa's lust for their bodies. In two days, 2–3 June 1885, 26 young men were burned to death at Namugongo, a short ride today from downtown Kampala.

Many more were hacked to death, speared, dismembered, torn alive by wild dogs or castrated before being burned. Others were given as gifts to pleasure Arab slave-masters and non-Christian chiefs.

The Protestants approached Bishop Livinhac of the White Fathers, urging that both religions join in a combined effort to stop the murders but Livinhac refused, saying it would make things worse. History often misjudges motives and I cannot say whether Livinhac was right or wrong.

However, Fr Lourdel, another White Father, believed in direct action. Against all protocol he broke through the guards and entered the audience hall to plead with the Kabaka. Further death sentences had already been pronounced and anyway I do not believe that Mwanga or his Katikkiro could be moved at this stage.

Many have since described the events at Namugongo and even tried to explain them. But no explanation and no length of time can wash away the blood that stains this page of history.

Both great Christian denominations remember. Pope Paul V1 canonised the Ugandan martyrs in 1964 and the Church of England has equally honoured its own – and even added three recent martyrs to the list – Archbishop Janani Luwum, Erinayo Oryema and Charles Ofumbi.

These three men did not die in 1885, instead they were martyred on the 17th February 1977, nearly 100 years later. All were mercilessly beaten and then riddled with bullets at the orders of Idi Amin.

Janani was only 55 when he was murdered and had been an outspoken critic of Amin's murderous regime. A statue now stands in his honour in Westminster Abbey.

Britain Takes Control

Public opinion was so inflamed in Britain by the atrocities in Uganda from 1885 to 1887 that it greatly facilitated the Imperial British East Africa Company in backing a rebellion against Mwanga and replacing him with his brother who had recently become a Muslim. This was a poor choice, and after a series of unsatisfactory Kabakas, the British restored Mwanga, but with much reduced powers and in a role where British hegemony was made absolutely clear.

Thus, when Lugard audaciously encamped on Kampala Hill in December 1890 and set up his maxim gun, Mwanga had no choice but to welcome him. Lugard's behaviour was unprecedented. Mwanga was in no position to object.

The British could now dictate terms and so, in 1894, they designated Uganda a British Protectorate. This determined the shape of things to come for many years.

On the plus side, Uganda now entered a phase of relative peace and prosperity and saw the practice of slavery abolished. On the down side the artificial creation of a single state, out of so many disparate and hostile tribes, sowed the seeds for future unrest and bloodshed. Furthermore, as with all colonists, the ultimate aim of the British was to strengthen their grip on central Africa, find an outlet for the goods they were manufacturing and exploit the local riches. In fairness, it must be admitted that there was a benevolence in British rule at a time when some other colonial powers were anything but benevolent.

Eventually the Christian churches became reconciled and even supported one another. Unfortunately, the peace that came into being between Christianity and Islam was more apparent than real and we can only hope that mutual respect and trust will win out in the end between these great religions.

APPENDIX 4

IDI AMIN DADA

Sow in Tears, Reap in a Whirlwind

Independence was a mixed blessing for many African countries. Those who benefitted were usually people already well established, well educated, politically astute and financially secure. Those who lost out were the minority tribes, the illiterate and the poor.

Development was concentrated on the major urban centres, while rural areas were neglected unless the current leader happened to come from a particular village. Power eventually corrupted the leaders of many new nations and as a result most of the upper classes became disenchanted or corrupt themselves. Ultimately no one trusted anyone.

The army always played a crucial role in keeping the ruler in power, but this support depended on giving the army special pay and special privileges. An elite loyal guard would be established and, of course, a special police with unlimited powers. Their job was to hunt down and eliminate anyone who spoke against the regime or who was alleged to disapprove of the way the country was run.

In practice this meant night-time raids, torture, rape, destruction and defilement of property and unbridled looting. It also turned neighbour against neighbour and even members of the same family against one another other.

Idi Amin destroyed Uganda exactly as outlined above.

Independent Uganda

A wave of independence from colonial rule swept Africa after Ghana declared itself a sovereign nation in 1957. Nigeria, Africa's sleeping giant, followed in 1960, and then it was Uganda's turn in 1962.

A new era had opened for Ugandans and there were high hopes that this relatively advanced African state would be a model of progress and peace for all emerging nations.

But the dreams that were born on 9th October 1962 were short lived. Within two years its first President, King Mutesa 11th was deposed and, after a succession of interim regimes, Milton Obote finally gained full control in 1966. As with all dictators Obote's rule was benign at first, but then gradually descended into a reign of terror.

Friendship is at best a fragile flower and can wither overnight where power is concerned. In Obote's case his friendship with Idi Amin – they had been partners in gold smuggling – did just that. While Obote was attending a Commonwealth Heads of Government Meeting in Singapore. Amin, the army man, seized power. Oboe's dictatorship had lasted just five years.

Idi Amin CBE
'Conqueror of the British Empire'

'No one can run faster than a bullet' (Idi Amin)

Clever, cunning, cruel, colourful, unpredictable, charismatic, take your pick, Amin was any and all of them. And you can add in cowardly, as his ultimate downfall demonstrated.

Initially, his accession to power in 1971 was greeted with jubilation. He had timed his coup perfectly taking advantage of Obote's absence and relying on the army to back him – after promising it special privileges should he succeed.

At this point too, not only the people of Uganda, but many in outside countries, including Israel, backed him, and he was internationally applauded for his statesman-like assertion that he would lead Uganda 'out of corruption, depression and slavery' and would 'organize a genuinely democratic civilian government'.

Amin's rise to power had been meteoric and much has been written about his personal charm, love for children, physical prowess and driving ambition. But more has been written about his sadistic cruelty, his need to humiliate others, his unpredictable moods, his paranoia and his total disregard for morality. For that is what the world really remembers.

Although he was first educated in a Catholic mission school, by the age of 15 he discarded that religion and embraced Sunni Islam. It was understandable that he should do so for his early upbringing as a member of the Kakwa tribe was far more Islamic than Christian. But his religion was only skin deep, and, once in power, he used it blatantly to woo Libya's Ghaddafi and the heads of other oil-rich Islamic states, after Western powers had become disenchanted with him. He further ingratiated himself with the dollar-rich oil states by denouncing his former ally Israel, destroying all synagogues in Uganda and expelling virtually all Jews.

He famously proclaimed that an Arab victory over Israel was inevitable, that he would send troops to help crush the Jews and that Goldameir would have to 'tuck up her knickers and run to Washington'. This kind of crude rhetoric was sweet music for anyone who hated Israel.

However, the Asians living in Uganda were an easier target.

Less than a year after seizing power, he expelled up to 100,000 of them including Muslim Asians. They were the backbone of the Ugandan economy but that counted for nothing as he knew he would gain even more popularity with the masses if he were seen to crush the wealthy. He did just that and 'generously' gave the expropriated properties to his followers. The unfortunate Asians were given 90 days to leave.

The rest of the world was now beginning to believe Amin when he pronounced that 'there is freedom of speech, but I cannot guarantee freedom after speech.' The UN watched shocked and horrified and did nothing.

For the next eight years, Amin ruled with increasing ruthlessness, all the while depending for his popularity on the masses, who admired his panache, his largesse and his humiliating treatment of the West.

However much Idi Amin Dada was cheered in public, the man who openly admired and copied Hitler was inevitably heading for a fall. Initially people were too afraid to do or say anything that might be considered remotely critical of him, but his public stock fell seriously after the dramatic rescue by Israeli commandos of hostages held in Entebbe.

Flight to Freedom

Palestinian freedom fighters had hijacked Air France flight 139 on 27th June 1976 and the plane now stood silent and empty on the runway at Entebbe. Its passengers were crowded under guard in the transit lounge awaiting their fate. The world held its breath waiting to see what would happen.

A week later, one of the most daring rescues in history took place when Israeli commandoes freed the hostages killing all the hijackers plus at least 20 Ugandan soldiers. Two hostages were accidentally shot. A third was shot by their Ugandan captors. Enraged by letting the Israelis snatch the bait from his trap, Amin ordered the execution of the entire civilian staff that was on duty that night in the airport.

The loss of face, the daring nature of operation and the widely known murder of innocent Ugandans by their own Government humiliated all Ugandans and made them look like idiots in the eyes of the world. Despite all Amin's propaganda, details of the rescue leaked out, and soon mutterings against him spread out from Kampala to the remotest corner of the land.

The Murder of Dora Bloch

People were actually more shocked and humiliated by an appalling sequel to the Israeli raid, which pushed Amin further into disgrace. This was the inexcusable murder of Dora Bloch.

Dora Bloch was a 75-year-old Israeli grandmother with a British passport who had been on flight AF-139. She had been taken hostage along with the others but got so ill in the terminal building – where they were all crowded together like animals – that two of the guards allowed her to be taken to Mulago Hospital for treatment. This was several hours before the Israeli paratroopers arrived.

Once Amin realised that he had been made look a fool, he had the old lady pulled out of her sick bed, driven out of Kampala and then riddled with bullets on the Jinja road. Her body was not returned to Israel until 1979.This ruthless murder, more than anything else, turned every decent person against Amin. Even his most ardent admirers no longer considered him a lovable buffoon.

Amin's Tunnel of Torture

On a recent visit to Kampala, three of us from the College of Surgeons in Ireland, Mary Leader, Clive Lee and myself, were given a tour of Amin's 'tunnel of torture'. It is in the grounds of his palace on Mengo Hill, between the right-hand side of the main building and a man-made lake. The opening is large enough to take several people side by side, and the stone floor dips sharply down into a dark interior. It was to this place that the secret police brought people suspected of criticising the regime.

God only knows how many were herded into that tunnel. Before entering, they were told to take off their shoes and leave them on the ground. 'This is because the floor of the tunnel is flooded with water and we want to save your shoes from damage.' They were assured everyone's shoes would be returned next day.

Most people did as asked, not suspecting the real reason for this strange request. A crack of a cane or a blow of a rifle butt encouraged the hesitant to do likewise. And then it seemed a sensible request, for the water got deeper and deeper as they moved down the tunnel until it reached above their ankles.

As the detainees were herded forward, their eyes became adjusted to the dim light and they saw a series of large empty rooms on their left-hand side. The rooms were barred off from the tunnel by thick metal bars each six inches apart. Solid steel doors were inserted into the metal fencing, one for each room. It suddenly became clear that these 'rooms' were in reality prison cells.

Up to 100 people were squashed into each cell and the doors then swung across and bolted for the night. Men cursed, women wept and children whimpered. It was stifling hot and there was no privacy. Indeed, there was not enough room for everyone to lie down on the damp stone floor.

There was no longer any doubt about their fate. Some scraped goodbye messages on the wall; others wrote their names using their own blood as ink. Just a few of the scrawls remain decipherable today and they cry out more loudly than any words can describe.

Bare electric bulbs were spaced on the wall of the tunnel facing these dungeon cells. They threw a soft orange glow on the puckered stone that glistened with moisture. Here and there thick black cables hung down from the roof and rested on to the floor below. The ends of the cables were not visible and to the casual observer they seemed to have no discernible purpose. But of course, those in the cells would soon discover their purpose.

Initially the shoeless victims were left in the dark and with no food or water; a squashed mass of human-ity, caged like animals in stench-filled darkness. A sleep-less night passed slowly and by dawn the prisoners were dazed and exhausted and obsessed by the thought of getting out of their dungeon cages. The jailers knew this. So in the morning they swung open the doors and walked off casually, knowing full well that people would dash for freedom.

Obviously, to escape, one had to make it to the tunnel entrance and face armed guards. But many had money and jewellery sequestered in their clothing and were confident that they could bribe their way out. Such a prospect was daunting but worth a try for desperate people. Once again, the guards had outwitted them. Dead bodies could be plundered at ease.

During the night, the floor of the tunnel had been flooded with salty water, perhaps to a depth of a six inches, so that it became a kind of river leading straight down to the lake. But this was no ordinary river. This time the cables had been activated so that they now became high-voltage bare-ended electric wires. Anyone who stepped out of a cell in bare feet would be electrocuted or savagely burnt.

The electrocuted, the half-dead and the senseless – after being relieved of anything worthwhile – were swept conveniently into the nearby lake. Here they made tasty meals for the local crocodiles or simply floated for days on the surface, bloated and distorted.

The only other time I have been so disgusted by the depravity of man was when I visited Auschwitz-Birkenau. We know Idi Amin admired Hitler. But it seems incredible that he descended with him to such black depths.

Idi Amin rates with the likes of Pol Pot, Gaddafi, Bokassa, Stalin, Hitler and a string of others whose names will forever burn in the book of Hell.

Tunnel Postscript

You couldn't build such a setup without the world knowing about it. So, overtly, the world was told that the tunnel and the underground bunkers were designed to house missiles and rockets which could be used if Kampala was attacked.

I understand that the Chinese built the complex, but whoever did, surely, they had no idea for what purpose Amin intended to use it.

The End of Amin

In 1979, Amin's implacable enemy, Julius Nyerere of Tanzania, finally succeeded in getting rid of him. The Tanzanian army together with Ugandan exiles invaded Uganda and, with defeat facing him, Amin fled to Saudi Arabia. He died in Jeddah in 2003. He was 78-years old. Few mourn his loss.

Post-Amin

In 1979, Obote was restored as President of Uganda. His second reign was even worse than his first one. Repression and death stalked the land. Things got worse when people thought they couldn't possibly get worse. But they did in 1983 when the Obote government launched Operation Bonanza, a military expedition that claimed up to 500,000 lives mostly of the Baganda and western Nilotic peoples. The people of Northern Uganda and freelance guerrillas supported Obote and the whole country was once again thrown into confusion and inter-tribal animosity. Anarchy threatened.

By now, Obote's own generals were completely disillusioned and deposed him in a *coup d'état* in July 1985. He was lucky to have escaped with his life and luckier still to receive sanctuary in Tanzania.

There followed a series of transient Presidents and

military rulers until finally Yoweri Museveni – an avowed anti-Obote activist – was elected President in January 1986, a post he still held in 2017.

Obote died in Johannesburg in 2005.

APPENDIX 5

BACKDROP TO THE BOSNIAN WAR

The history of the Balkans is complicated and difficult to condense into a few paragraphs. It is a litany of invasions and of bloody internecine wars, dominated by ethnic and religious fanaticism. It is a long history, where the sophisticated and the barbaric go hand in hand. It is a history in which empires have come and gone, sometimes leaving an indelible imprint on civilisation, sometimes vanishing without a trace.

In the following pages, we skimp through the recent history of this intriguing part of the world in the hope that it will give us a better understanding of the terrible war that took place there between 1992 and 1995. Like other wars there was a long lead up before the open conflagration in 1992 and, in a similar way, the ceasefire of 1995 did not signify a sudden end to hostilities but was rather a defining moment after which an uneasy peace gradually settled on the land.

After 400 years of Ottoman domination, most of the Balkans became part of the Austro-Hungarian Empire in 1878. This was a situation resented and resisted by all the local factions. Yet, despite repeated ambushes and reprisals, things remained so until 1918 and the end of the First World War. With the defeat of the Axis powers, the people of the Balkans were amalgamated into a single state that would be called Yugoslavia.

The major groups within the new state were Croats, Serbs, Slovenes and Bosniaks. Unfortunately, Yugoslavia was united in name only, for the struggle for dominance between the four groups caused recurrent and often violent clashes.

One major faction was the Ustaše, a fiercely fascist Roman Catholic militia, whose aim was to establish a Greater Croatia and in the process exterminate Serbs, Jews, Romanies and moderate Croats.

The other major faction, the Chetniks, aimed to establish a Greater Serbia. The Chetniks were a long-established part of the regular army but mainly consisted of gangs of ruthless Serbs who struck terror everywhere they went.

So it was inevitable that these two forces, which had diametrically opposite visions for the future of the Balkans, should clash and clash violently.

World War II (WWII) and the Nazi invasion brought further unrest and devastation to an already war-torn country, and threw strange bedfellows together.

At first both the Ustaše and the Chetniks collaborated with the Nazis. They both wanted to use the Nazis to further their own aims and were prepared to do anything to achieve this. Soon, however, they found that the Nazis would not tolerate independent actions by either group unless it strengthened Nazi control. So they turned against them, betrayed them and eventually ambushed them. Nonetheless, at no stage did the Ustaše or the Chetniks renounce their hatred for each other.

Into this mix came a third local group, the Partisans. Marshal Josip Tito, an avowed Communist – but never a complete lackey of Moscow – led these. In many ways, he controlled or suppressed the warring factions and his partisans certainly gave the Germans – and the Chetniks – a rough time.

After WWII he broke with Stalin and introduced a progressive and moderate form of communism into Yugoslavia. He also became a frequent visitor to the West where he was warmly welcomed but where mutual trust was completely lacking. He seemed to steer a course half way between Communism and Capitalism. He wooed both but never kowtowed to either. As a result, neither side trusted him completely. However, he did manage to keep Yugoslavia relatively calm.

After Tito's death in 1980, old rivalries flared up once more. Things gradually deteriorated over the next ten years and no one was surprised when both Slovenia and Croatia seceded from the war-torn country in 1991.

At this time Bosnia, like Montenegro and Kosovo, was still essentially a part of Serbia. But in view of anti-Bosniak events in Croatia and Slovenia, the Bosnians decided to hold a referendum and promptly declared their independence the following year – 1992. The European Union – with unusual haste – recognised the State of BiH within months.

The Serbs living in BiH were angry at being ignored and wanted no part of the new State. So they established a *de facto* Republica Srpska, with its capital in Banja Luka. They looked to Belgrade – the Serbian capital – for support, and this was given without hesitation.

The Bosnian War was now about to start in earnest, despite many fruitless albeit sometimes valiant efforts to avert it.

In short it can be said that the Bosnian War was fought because Serbs and Croats living in Bosnia wanted to annex 'Bosnian territory' each for themselves.

Historians will surely throw up their hands in despair at such a superficial analysis and show that there were far more elements in bringing the Balkan unrest to crisis point. However, they will not quibble when I say that the subsequent conflagration brought out the worst and the best in people, with depravity beyond description and bravery beyond belief displayed by both sides.

EVIL DOINGS IN THE BALKANS

Medjugorje: Massacres not Miracles

By 1992, the little miracle town was fast becoming a centre for hatred and bloodshed rather than for prayer. Tensions between Croats, Serbs and Bosniaks had always existed in and around Medjugorje and now came to a head. Since these three groups are broadly speaking adherents of Christianity, Eastern Orthodoxy and Islam, it is easy to see why many blame religious fanatics for the atrocities that were soon to take place. No one side is totally at fault. All were wrong. All acted in the name of nationalism, patriotism and religious conviction.

Nor should we forget a fourth group, the true Communists, who systematically murdered members of all religions, but who seemed to have an especial hatred for the Franciscans.

It is worth recalling specific examples of the kind of horrors ordinary peaceful people had to endure even before 1992. My first example concerns a Serbian Orthodox monastery at Žitomislić near Medjugorje. This monastery, dedicated to the Annunciation of the Virgin Mary, has stood there since 1566 and was always a place of prayer. It was also a place of welcome for travelling pilgrims and its famous library was a haven for scholars from all over the world. On June 21 1941, armed fanatical Roman

Catholic Croatian nationalists, looted the monastery and, after torturing the monks, buried seven of them alive. Two months later – nor far from Medjugorje – the Ustaše (Croatian fascists) murdered almost 2,000 unarmed Serb civilians, throwing many – while still alive – into a deep pit at Golubinka. This became known as the Golubinka Pit massacre. Fifty years on, in 1992, the Croatian Defense Council (HVO) completed the grisly work in a manner that can only be compared to that of the Germans in Warsaw during WWII. They razed the monastery to the ground with bulldozers and burned down the magnificent library with its many treasures and its priceless ancient Turkish manuscripts.

Later the scattered stones would be carefully gathered and the monastery slowly rebuilt. Thus, by 2005, when I first saw it, the buildings and church had regained some of their former splendour, but locals told me it would never be the same.

However, all was not one sided. Unfortunately, when members of one group slaughtered members of another the reprisals were excessive and often barbaric in nature. My second example concerns the massacre at Vokovar.

A year before the HVO destruction of Žitomislić, the eastern Croatian town of Vukovar was besieged by the Serbian (syn. Yugoslavian) army.

The town, noted for its lovely baroque architecture, eventually surrendered but no quarter was given and every building was razed to the ground.

Destruction was so complete that people later called it the 'Croatian Stalingrad'. The massacre of any prisoners taken was savage, terrifying and merciless. It is hard to be certain of numbers but – for sure – at least 300 POWs were beaten for hours and then shot in groups of twenty, after which they were dumped into pits. Locals report that over 3,000 Croatian soldiers were slaughtered either during or after the fall of the city.

Ironically, Vukovar could have been relieved by the Croatian army had their President Tubman given the order. But he did not do so on the grounds that he could not spare soldiers from other operations. Many hotly deny this.

Srebrenica July 1995

The only atrocity that remains in public consciousness outside the Balkans now is the massacre in Srebrenica. Here 8000 Bosniaks – mostly of Muslim men and boys – were murdered in July 2005. This was carried out by elements of the army of the Republic of Srpska (VRS) under General Ratko Mladić. Much of the blame for this savagery must be attributed to autonomous paramilitary groups such as the Serbian Scorpions. Paramilitary militias were prominent on all sides in the Bosnian War and were feared by everyone because of their utter ruthlessness and disregard for normal moral principles. I have no doubt that Mladić – the 'butcher of Bosnia' – co-operated with them, but I also suspect that he merely turned a blind eye to their behaviour rather than give the direct order himself.

Today we remember Srebrenica with shame, not least because the UN Dutchbat, strictly obeying their orders of non-interference, stood by, while the murders – afterwards labelled genocide – took place. I was in Sarajevo at the time and was among those who dismissed the news that was seeping out as exaggeration and propaganda. It was only much later, when I had returned to Ireland, that I learned the dreadful truth of what happened that fateful day.

APPENDIX 7

ASSASSINATION OF FERDINAND AND SOPHIE

The crumbling Austro-Hungarian empire controlled most of the Balkans up to the Great War of 1914–1918. Their rule was resented and actively opposed by many nationalistic groups but no more so than in Sarajevo where a group of nationalistic young men plotted against the oppressor. An ideal opportunity to strike a blow for freedom came on the occasion of the visit to Sarajevo of Archduke Ferdinand, heir to the Hapsburg throne in Austria, and his young wife Sophie in 1914.

Can I remind you briefly of the sad events of 28th June 1914? The royal party had narrowly escaped an earlier assassination attempt that Sunday morning and, instead of abandoning their visit, decided to make a surprise call on those injured in the failed attempt. They would drive to the hospital using an unscheduled route. Everyone approved of this.

As the cavalcade drove west along Appel Quay and approached the Latin Bridge, the driver slowed and mistakenly turned right into Franz Joseph Strasse instead of driving straight on.

By chance, nineteen-year-old Gavrilo Princip was standing outside Schiller's food shop on the corner. Young Princip was one of a group of Slavic zealots who wanted to throw off the yoke of the Austro-Hungarian Empire and had been involved in planning the failed attempt to kill the Archduke earlier that day. Now, purely by accident, he suddenly came face to face with the royal couple. He did not hesitate. He shot twice.

The first bullet entered Sophie's abdomen and she died in her husband's arms; the second struck the Archduke in the neck and he died shortly afterwards in hospital. Sophie was expecting their first child at the time. Some say the Archduke called 'Sophie' as he fell across her and that he died before reaching hospital. Other accounts insist he was still alive when he reached hospital.

While the exact sequence of events immediately surrounding the death of Franz and Sophie varies from commentator to commentator, all agree on what happened to Gavrilo Princip. Within moments of the shooting security guards jumped on the gunman and bundled him to the ground. He was dazed and bruised by the time he was fully apprehended and dragged into a prison cell. The whole incident provoked international outrage and black edged commemorative postage stamps were subsequently issued in Vienna carrying the image of the beautiful young heiress and the archduke. But more importantly Gavrilo had unwittingly set off a series of events that would lead to WWI, the bloodiest war in history.

Because he was twenty seven days short of his twentieth birthday he was given a life sentence (twenty years) rather than being hanged. Hanging would have been preferable. He was treated abominably in prison and he wasted away from rampant TB, insufficient food and constant mistreatment. He tried to kill himself on more than one occasion but always failed. Eventually, in April

1918, he passed away, unheralded and uncared for. He weighed just over six stone (80 lbs).

Gavrilo was buried secretly, but a Serb soldier knew the location of his grave and so, many years later, his body was found and reinterred in St Mark's cemetery in Sarajevo. Many Serbs revere him today as a hero.

Franz Joseph Strasse has since been renamed Zelenih beretki and Appel Quay is now Obala Kulina bana, but the Latin bridge is called 'Princip's Bridge' by many of the older people. They still speak in hushed tones of that June day in 1914 and of the nervous youth who happened to be there stood and ended three young lives – a fourth if you include his own.

Such were my thoughts as I stood beside the small plaque that commemorates these events and looked across that same Latin Bridge and beyond to the hills, from which hostile guns were again spewing death and destruction on this benighted city.